MULTISKILLING:

Respiratory Care

FOR THE HEALTH CARE PROVIDER

ACKNOWLEDGMENTS

Appreciation is expressed to the following practitioners and educators for their critical reviews of the manuscript:

Ken Bretl, College of DuPage, Glen Ellyn, IL
Diana Luder, Northeast Wisconsin Technical College, Greenbay, WI
Theresa Piurkowsky, Trident Technical College, Charleston, SC
Joseph Ross, Baltimore City Community College, Baltimore, MD
Ruth P. Thompson, West Kentucky Technical College, Paducah, KY

MULTISKILLING:

Respiratory Care

FOR THE HEALTH CARE PROVIDER

James R. Sills,
MEd, CPFT, RRT
Rock Valley College, Rockford, IL

Beverly M. Kovanda
PhD, MS, MT (ASCP), CLP (NCA)
Series Editor

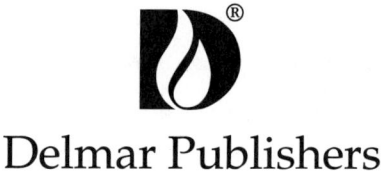

Delmar Publishers

an International Thomson Publishing company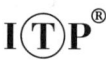

Albany • Bonn • Boston • Cincinnati • Detroit • London • Madrid
Melbourne • Mexico City • New York • Pacific Grove • Paris • San Francisco
Singapore • Tokyo • Toronto • Washington

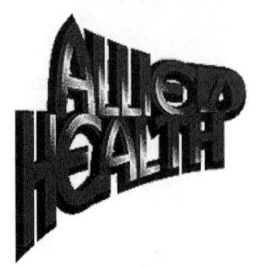
Cover Design: Scott Keidong's Image Enterprises
Delmar Staff
Publisher: Susan Simpfenderfer
Acquisitions Editor: Dawn Gerrain
Developmental Editor: Marjorie A. Bruce
Project Editor: Brooke Graves/Graves Editorial Service
Team Assistant: Sandra Bruce

Art and Design Coordinator: Vincent S. Berger
Production Coordinator: John Mickelbank
Marketing Manager: Katherine Slezak
Marketing Coordinator: Glenna Stanfield
Editorial Assistant: Donna L. Leto

COPYRIGHT © 1998
By Delmar Publishers
a division of International Thomson Publishing Inc.

The ITP logo is a trademark under license.

Printed in the United States of America

For more information, contact:

Delmar Publishers
3 Columbia Circle, Box 15015
Albany, New York 12212-5015

International Thomson Publishing Europe
High Holborn
Berkshire House 168-173
London, WC1V 7AA
England

Thomas Nelson Australia
102 Dodds Street
South Melbourne, 3205
Victoria, Australia

Nelson Canada
1120 Birchmount Road
Scarborough, Ontario
Canada, M1K 5G4

International Thomson Editores
Campos Eliseos 385, Piso 7
Col Polanco
11560 Mexico D F Mexico

International Thomson Publishing GmbH
Konigswinterer Strasse 418
53227 Bonn
Germany

International Thomson Publishing Asia
221 Henderson Road
#05-10 Henderson Building
Singapore 0315

International Thomson Publishing—Japan
Hirakawacho Kyowa Building, 3F
2-2-1 Hirakawacho
Chiyoda-ku, Tokyo 102
Japan

1 2 3 4 5 6 7 8 9 10 XXX 03 02 01 00 99 98 97

Library of Congress Cataloging-in-Publication Data

Sills. James R.
    Multiskilling : respiratory care for the health care provider /
James R. Sills.
    p. cm.
    Includes index.
    ISBN 0–7668–0075–X–
    1. Respiratory therapy. 2. Nurses' aides. 3. Cardiopulmonary
system—Physiology. 4. Cardiopulmonary system—Diseases—Nursing.
I. Title.
    [DNLM: 1. Respiratory Therapy. WB 342 S584m 1998]
RC735.I5S577 1998
616.2'0046—dc21
DNLM/DLC
for Library of Congress   97-42387
                                                                  CIP

The Multiskilling for Health Care Providers series consists of the *Patient Care: Basic Skills for the Health Care Provider* core text and many separate modular texts. The Multiskilling series offers a comprehensive vision of the diversity and many implications of multiskilling, whether in an acute care setting, home care, hospice, ambulatory setting, long-term care facility, or physician's office. The core text and module subjects have been identified through research as key topics in multiskilling and patient care training across the nation.

The framework for this series is found in the historic evolution of multiskilling, the National Health Care Skill Standards, and 13 years of personal experience in developing academic material and successfully training thousands of multiskilled health care providers in a multitude of nursing and allied health skill areas. The concept referred to as *multiskilling, crosstraining,* and (more recently) *patient care skills* began to gain national awareness in the mid-1980s, as pressures for cost containment in health care intensified. Institutions began to focus on more efficient use of personnel for economic survival. The implications of managed care are far-reaching.

In 1994, the National Health Care Skill Standards were developed through a national collaborative effort of health care organizations, professional organizations, schools, and colleges of higher education. By implementing these standards, we can more effectively serve the needs of a diverse client population and maintain quality care, while increasing the efficiency of staff utilization. Health care costs can be contained; the new technology, which is changing how and where health care is delivered, can be prudently applied. We believe that the skill standards are important and so their intent has been incorporated into the entire series.

The core text, *Patient Care: Basic Skills for the Health Care Provider,* meets the OBRA requirements for basic patient care skills. These skills are required of every health care provider who undertakes client care, regardless of the institutional setting or professional affiliation.

We believe that the core-text-plus-modules concept is the only rational approach to meeting the vastly different academic and training needs in multiskilling, as we re-engineer careers in all health care settings. The modules are flexible, well written, and academically sound. The modular approach is cost-effective. A health care worker's skills can be developed based upon individual goals, institutional needs for retraining, or specific career development. Colleges, hospitals, other health care agencies, technical and career schools, and "tech prep" programs need only purchase the modules that address their unique, customized academic and training needs. Because multiskilling is market-driven, other modules continue to be developed as health care needs are identified and evolve.

The modules are written by credentialed experts in each content area and multiskilling education. They have identified essential and appropriate nursing and allied health skills that can be accurately and safely performed by nonprofessionals to enhance the quality of patient care.

The depth of theory and skills in each module goes beyond other texts, which are usually written from the perspective of one profession rather than by specialists in each identifiable allied health and nursing area. We believe that this principle provides a stronger basis for instruction and facilitates a higher level of quality patient care.

The material in each module is organized in a clear, concise, straightforward manner to make learning easier, because health care institutions are demanding shorter—but intensified—training periods. The pedagogical features enhance retention and simplify learning.

We believe that the Multiskilling series combines the knowledge, experience, successes, and expertise of all of the authors. It provides the tools and flexibility to custom-design a curriculum that truly meets worker/student professional goals, augments valuable skills, and strengthens employability, not only now but as we prepare for the 21st century.

Beverly M. Kovanda, Ph.D., M.S., M.T. (ASCP), C.L.P. (NCA)
Coordinator/Professor
Multicompetency Health Technology

DELMAR'S MULTISKILLING SERIES

Patient Care: Basic Skills for the Health Care Provider
Multiskilling: Advanced Patient Care Skills for the Health Care Provider
Multiskilling: Phlebotomy Collection Procedures for the Health Care Provider
Multiskilling: Electrocardiography for the Health Care Provider
Multiskilling: Respiratory Care for the Health Care Provider
Multiskilling: Point of Care Testing-Capillary Puncture for the Health Care Provider

Modules Coming Soon:
Multiskilling: Waived Lab Testing for the Health Care Provider
Multiskilling: Team Building for the Health Care Provider
Multiskilling: Health Unit Coordinator for the Health Care Provider
Multiskilling: Physical Therapy/Rehabilitation Aide for the Health Care Provider
Multiskilling: Dietetic Aide for the Health Care Provider
Multiskilling: Basic Life Support for the Health Care Provider

Table of CONTENTS

PREFACE

This book introduces the functioning of the lungs and heart, related systems, common diseases that affect the cardiopulmonary system, and frequently seen treatment methods for these diseases. As health care evolves, it is important that we all understand what other health care workers are doing and, in some cases, be able to perform some of each other's duties. You are part of a health care team and you will be assisting the respiratory care practitioner (RCP) or registered nurse (RN) in the care of these patients. You may also find that you are expected to perform some basic respiratory care treatments.

This text is written to help educate you on how to perform these treatments. However, simply reading this book will not adequately prepare you for the important things that you will do. Experienced practitioners will also be teaching you in the classroom, laboratory, and clinical settings. Checkoffs of the steps involved in safely performing a given procedure are included at the end of the book. They will probably be used as part of the educational process. Depending on your place of employment, these checkoffs may be modified. Additionally, your employer may choose not to have you perform some listed procedures. Throughout this text, caution statements are placed if there is a possibility of a patient being harmed or reacting badly to a procedure. Always be on the lookout for problems with your patients. If you notice a problem or have any questions, get help from the physician, RN, or RCP.

Because health care is always changing with new ideas and equipment, it is important that you welcome change and remain anxious to learn. The vocation of health care is, I think, the most noble of all. It will offer you many rewards as you work to help your patients get better and lead productive lives.

CHAPTER 1

Basic Cardiopulmonary Anatomy and Physiology

- **cardiac:** *concerning or involving the heart*
- **pulmonary:** *concerning or involving the lungs*
- **oxygen:** *a tasteless, odorless, colorless gas essential for respiration in humans and most forms of animal life. Earth's atmosphere is composed of almost 21% oxygen. Oxygen supports combustion and is highly active in many chemical reactions*
- **carbon dioxide:** *a colorless, odorless gas produced by the oxidation of carbon. Carbon dioxide, as a product of cell respiration, is carried by the blood to the lungs to be exhaled. Only trace amounts are found in the atmosphere*
- **diffuse:** *become widely spread, such as through a membrane of fluid. Diffusion is the process in which a substance, such as a gas, moves from an area of higher concentration to an area of lower concentration, resulting in an even distribution of the substance. No energy is required*
- **tissue:** *a collection of similar cells acting together to perform a particular function*
- **cell:** *the fundamental unit of all living tissue. A human cell consists of nucleus, cytoplasm, and organelles surrounded by a thin membrane*
- **metabolism:** *the total of all chemical processes that take place in living organisms, resulting in growth, generation of energy, elimination of wastes, and other bodily functions as they relate to the distribution of nutrients after digestion*
- **acid:** *a compound that yields hydrogen ions (H^+) when dissociated in solution. Acids have chemical properties essentially opposite to those of bases*
- **exhale (past tense, exhaled):** *to breathe out or to let out the breath*

OVERVIEW

The multiskilled entry-level health care worker (often called a patient care technician or PCT) must have a strong understanding of how the body functions. You must know normal anatomy (structure) and physiology (function) of the body before you can understand how illness or injury can disrupt normal functions. Depending on the patient's problem, treatments are given to return the body to healthy operation.

After the central nervous system, no other organ system is more important to a person's life and health than the cardiopulmonary system. This is because the heart (**cardiac** system) and lungs (**pulmonary** system) do two critically important things. First, they take the life-sustaining gas **oxygen** (O_2) into the body. Second, they remove the waste product gas **carbon dioxide** (CO_2) from the body. Oxygen is vital for life. A person who is deprived of it for just 4 to 6 minutes will suffer irreversible, permanent brain damage or even death. The lungs are designed to bring the oxygen in the air we breathe into close contact with blood so that the oxygen will **diffuse** into the blood. The heart pumps this oxygenated blood throughout the body. The oxygen then diffuses from the blood into **tissues** and individual **cells** to continue vital chemical processes. The body's **metabolism** is designed to use food (carbohydrates, fats, and proteins) and oxygen. Without the constant supply of oxygen, metabolism quickly slows down and then completely stops.

When the body has adequate supplies of oxygen and food, it produces three waste products. Two of these, urine and feces, must occasionally be eliminated from the body. The gas carbon dioxide is the third waste product. It must constantly be removed by the lungs. Carbon dioxide is produced by every living cell. From the cells it diffuses into the blood as the oxygen diffuses from the blood into the cells. The heart then pumps the deoxygenated (high carbon dioxide and low oxygen) blood back to the lungs. There the carbon dioxide is exhaled and new, oxygen-rich, fresh air is inhaled. Failure to remove the carbon dioxide results in chemical reactions that produce **acid.** If the levels of carbon dioxide and acid become too high, the person's metabolism is disrupted. This can ultimately lead to death.

Both the intake of oxygen and the removal of carbon dioxide require continuous breathing and circulation of the blood. The lungs and heart and all related breathing and circulatory structures work together as the cardiopulmonary system to perform this vital function. The anatomy and physiology briefly described in this chapter show the elegance of how the system operates. As will be seen in Chapter 2, many diseases can affect one or more parts of the cardiopulmonary system. Chapter 3 includes some of the treatments that are used to help patients with lung and/or heart disease.

PULMONARY SYSTEM

The pulmonary system is designed to enable the atmospheric gas oxygen to be brought into the body and the waste gas carbon dioxide to be removed from the body. For this to happen, a series of connected events must take place. The nervous system must sense the presence or absence of these gases in the body. Nerve signals must be sent to the muscles of breathing. Contraction of these muscles of breathing expands the lungs, pulling air in through the airways and into the lungs. After the lungs have been filled with fresh gas, the breathing muscles relax and the chest and lungs return to their resting positions. This causes part of the air in the lungs to be **exhaled.** These connected steps make up breathing and are covered in the first part of this chapter. Other important steps involved in moving oxygen into the body and carbon dioxide out of the body are done by the heart, circulatory system, and blood. They are discussed later in this chapter.

Upper Airway

The upper airway is made up of three areas: the nose, the mouth or oral cavity, and the **pharynx.** Together they are the outermost connection of the lungs to the atmosphere and world. The upper airway does five things:

1. Air from the atmosphere flows in through it and is humidified and adjusted to body temperature.
2. Waste gas from the body and lungs flows out through it.
3. It filters larger foreign particles out of the air so that they do not reach the lower airways and lungs.
4. Speech is formed in it.
5. The senses of taste and smell come from it.

The Nose

The nose is the main passageway for gases into and out of the lungs. It also conditions or prepares the inspired air, before that air reaches the lungs, in three ways:

1. Filters it to trap and remove dust, pollen, and other particulates
2. Adjusts the air temperature to body temperature
3. Humidifies the air so that it is not drying to the lungs.

The outer part of the nose is made up of skin, cartilage, and bone. Air enters through two nostrils or *nares*. About half of the inspired air goes into each nostril. A structure called the *nasal septum* internally divides the nose into left and right chambers. A moist, **mucous membrane** lines the two nasal passages and extends through the mouth to the smallest airways of the lungs. The air that enters each nostril then passes over the set of three **conchae** or **turbinates** found on that side (Figure 1-1). The turbinates are the main structures that filter, adjust the temperature, and humidify the inspired air. Some air may also enter the nasal **sinuses** (Figure 1-2). When we speak, voice quality is modified

■ *pharynx:* the throat, a tubular structure that extends from the back of the mouth and nasal passages to the esophagus and trachea. The pharynx serves as the passageway for the respiratory and digestive tracts and changes shape to allow the formation of various vocal sounds

■ *mucous membrane:* any one of four major kinds of thin sheets of tissue that cover or line various parts of the body that open to the outside. Mucous membranes secrete protective mucus and line the mouth, respiratory passages, digestive tube, and genitourinary tract

■ *concha* (plural, *conchae*): a shell-shaped structure found in the nasal passage. One of three folds of tissue in each nasal passage that increase its surface area for filtration, humidification, and temperature adjustment of inhaled air

■ *turbinate:* a scroll-shaped structure found in the nasal passage. See concha

■■ **Hint:** *Plug one nostril and inhale. Then do the same on the other side. Unless you have a head cold, allergies, or deviated septum, you should be able to breathe through both sides.* ■■

■ *sinuses* (singular, *sinus*): a cavity or channel, such as a cavity in bone, a dilated channel for venous blood, or one permitting the escape of purulent material

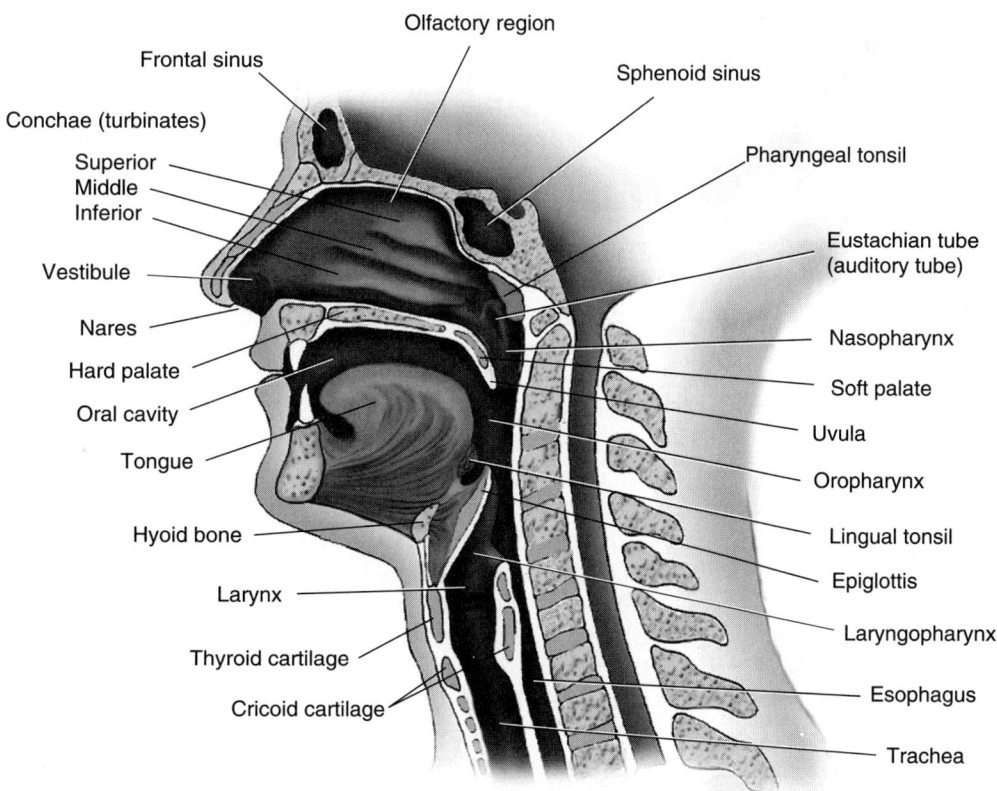

Figure 1-1 The major structures of the upper airway

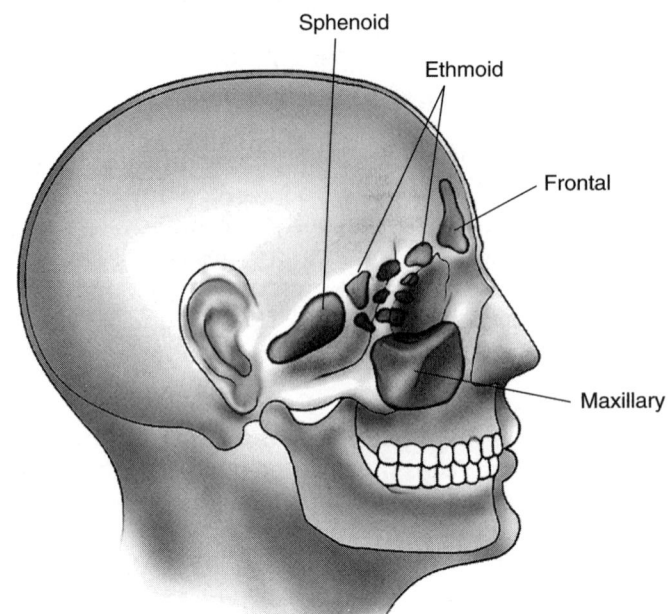

Sphenoid

Ethmoid

Frontal

Maxillary

Figure 1-2 The four sets of nasal sinuses, as seen from the right side

■ **olfactory:** *of or pertaining to the sense of smell*

■ **eustachian tube:** *a tube, lined with mucous membrane, that joins the nasopharynx and the middle ear cavity, allowing equalization of the air pressure in the middle ear with atmospheric pressure*

■ **nasopharynx:** *the uppermost of the three regions of the throat, or pharynx, situated behind the nose and extending from the posterior nares to the level of the soft palate*

■ **oropharynx:** *the middlemost of the three regions of the throat, or pharynx, situated behind the tongue and uvula*

■ **Hint:** *Seeing a patient lying in bed and gasping for air through an open mouth indicates real distress. Get help!* ■

■ **lymphatic system:** *a vast, complex network of capillaries, thin vessels, valves, ducts, nodes, and organs that helps to protect and maintain the internal fluid environment of the entire body by producing, filtering, and moving lymph fluid and producing various blood cells*

by the air moving through the turbinates and sinuses. The sense of smell comes from the **olfactory** region. Sniffing brings a small amount of air into the olfactory region and holds it there to increase the sense of smell. A **eustachian tube** (auditory tube) connects each inner ear with atmospheric pressure. This is important for pressure adjustment as you dive under water or fly in an airplane. The hard palate and soft palate separate the nasal passages from the oral cavity. Bone is found in the hard palate, but the soft palate tissues are flexible. The soft palate ends in the uvula (Figures 1-1 and 1-3). Both nasal passages come together in back of the turbinates in an area called the **nasopharynx.** It joins the **oropharynx** in the back of the oral cavity. The uvula bends up to separate the nasopharynx and oropharynx during such activities as swallowing, sucking, and blowing out.

The Mouth or Oral Cavity

The mouth acts as an air passage for breathing when the nasal passages cannot. If you have ever had a bad head cold, you know what it is like to have to breathe through your mouth! Nasal surgery or injury may also require a person to mouth breathe. During heavy exercise it is also most effective to breathe through the mouth.

The oral cavity is covered by the soft tissue of the lips and cheeks. The teeth are used for chewing food and are firmly anchored into bones. The maxilla is the bone of the upper jaw and the lower jaw bone is called the mandible. Strong muscles hold the mandible to the skull and are used for biting and chewing. The base of the mouth is made up of the tongue and related soft structures. The tongue is used for speech, eating, and the sense of taste. The lingual and palatine tonsils are part of the **lymphatic system** (Figures 1-1 and 1-3). Sometimes the tonsils are surgically removed if they have been chronically infected and are enlarged. The oropharynx, often referred to as the *throat,* is the back of the oral cavity. The oropharynx connects with the nasopharynx, as covered earlier, and the lower airways, which are discussed next.

The Lower Airways

The lower airways extend from the back of the oral cavity/oropharynx to the lung tissues. The main airway is a single tube that splits apart to go to each lung.

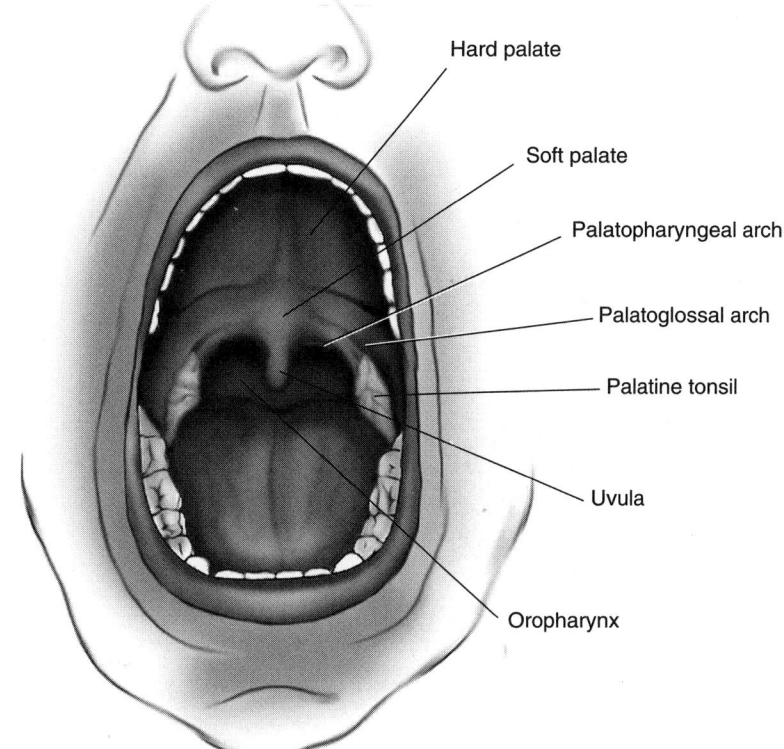

Hard palate

Soft palate

Palatopharyngeal arch

Palatoglossal arch

Palatine tonsil

Uvula

Oropharynx

Figure 1-3   The major structures of the oral cavity or mouth

■ *larynx:* the organ of voice that is part of the air passage connecting the pharynx with the trachea

■ *trachea:* a nearly cylindrical tube in the neck, composed of cartilage and membrane, that extends from the larynx into the chest, where it divides into two bronchi. The trachea allows air to move to the lungs

■ *vocal cords:* two bands of yellow, strong, elastic tissue in the larynx enclosed by membranes called vocal folds. When air passes over them, they vibrate and produce sounds

■ *glottis:* a slit-like opening between the vocal cords

■ *epiglottis:* the cartilaginous structure that overhangs the larynx like a lid and prevents food and liquids from entering the larynx and trachea while swallowing

■ *aspiration:* the act of inhaling food, liquids, or foreign matter into the airways and/or lungs

■ *esophagus:* a muscular canal extending from the pharynx to the stomach. Food and liquids pass through it to the stomach.

■ *Valsalva maneuver:* any forced expiratory effort against a closed airway, such as when an individual holds the breath and tightens the muscles in a concerted, strenuous effort to move a heavy object, deliver a baby, or empty the bowel

■ *tracheobronchial tree:* an anatomic complex that includes the trachea, the bronchi, and the bronchial tubes. It conveys air to and from the lungs and is a primary structure in ventilation

From there, the airway to each lung divides again and again so that air is directed to smaller and smaller portions of lung tissue.

The Larynx

The top part of the lower airways is the **larynx.** It is located between the oropharynx and the **trachea** (Figure 1-1). The larynx is where speech originates, and all air passes through it. Sound is created by the movement of air between and over the **vocal cords** (Figure 1-4). The vocal cords are made up of strong, elastic ligaments. Normally they are partially open so that air can move easily between them. This opening is called the **glottis.** During speech and singing, muscles open and close the vocal cords to create lower or higher pitched sounds. The tongue, lips, and oral and nasal passages are used to alter the sounds into words.

Besides the creation of sound, the larynx has two other important jobs. First, it fits together with the **epiglottis** to protect the lower airways from the **aspiration** of liquids, solid food, or foreign matter. During swallowing, the larynx is pulled up and the epiglottis covers the glottis (Figures 1-1 and 1-4). Normally this prevents anything from entering the trachea. The food is directed down the **esophagus** into the stomach. Probably everyone has experienced a small amount of food or drink going "down the wrong pipe." Usually this happens when you are talking or laughing while eating. The presence of food in the trachea stimulates a strong cough to blow it out. The second important function of the larynx is its voluntary closing during exhalation. This is called the **Valsalva maneuver.** During it, the vocal cords close completely against a forced exhalation. The resulting buildup of pressure within the lungs also pushes down on the abdominal contents. This increased pressure helps with a strong cough, lifting a heavy object, a bowel movement, or childbirth.

The Tracheobronchial Tree

The **tracheobronchial tree** starts at the lower end of the larynx and subdivides repeatedly as the airways penetrate to the smallest parts of the lungs. The

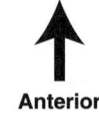

Anterior

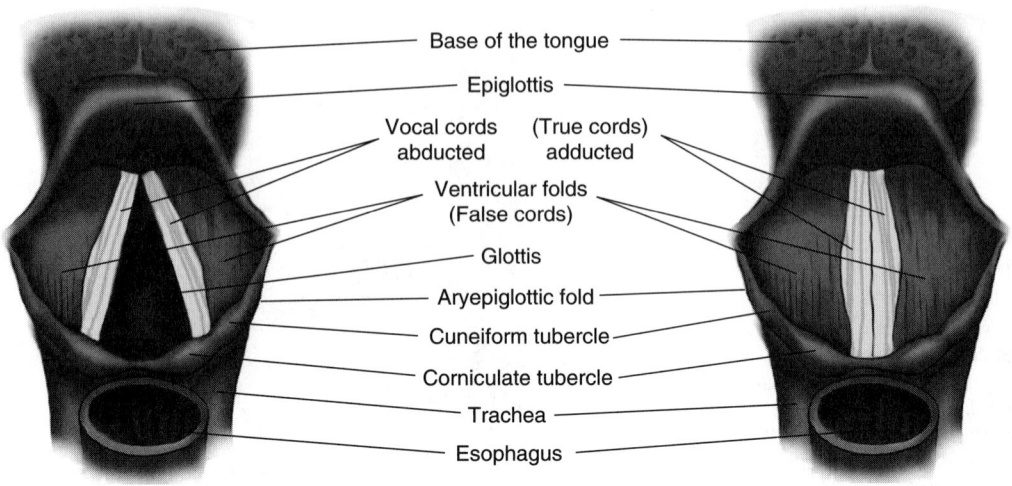

Base of the tongue

Epiglottis

Vocal cords   (True cords)
abducted   adducted

Ventricular folds
(False cords)

Glottis

Aryepiglottic fold

Cuneiform tubercle

Corniculate tubercle

Trachea

Esophagus

Figure 1-4   The structures of the larynx, as seen from above

■ *conducting zone: the airways that do not contact alveoli and through which no gas is exchanged. See* dead space

■ *dead space (anatomic dead space): the volume in the trachea, bronchi, and air passages containing air that does not reach the alveoli during inspiration*

■ *respiratory zone: the airways that contact alveoli and through which gas is exchanged*

■ *alveolar sac: an air sac at one of the terminal cavities of lung tissue. It is composed of 15 to 20 individual alveoli*

■ *alveoli: small outpouchings of walls of alveolar space through which gas exchange takes place between alveolar air and pulmonary capillary blood*

■ *centimeter (cm): a unit of length in the metric system of measurement. One inch is 2.54 cm long*

phrase *tracheobronchial tree* is used because, much like an actual tree, there is a main supporting structure (trunk/trachea) which then divides repeatedly (branches/bronchi) before reaching the area where gases are exchanged (leaves/alveoli). Altogether there are between 24 and 27 different branchings of the airways. (See Table 1-1.) With each branching the airways become progressively shorter and smaller in diameter. Each splitting of the airway is called a *generation* or *order*. The first nine generations of airways are supported by incomplete rings of cartilage. The cartilage gives the airways strength to retain their shape for airflow yet allows them flexibility. This is necessary because the lungs and airways must bend with lung expansion and contraction during breathing. The next 10 generations do not contain any cartilage. These very small airways are supported by spiral muscle fibers (also called smooth muscle) and the surrounding lung tissue. These first 19 generations of airways are often called the **conducting zone.** This means that they conduct air between the atmosphere and the lung tissue. No actual gas exchange takes place within the conducting zone airways.

The term **dead space** may be used to describe the conducting zone airways. Dead space also refers to that part of the breath that does not reach the alveoli to participate in gas exchange. With each inspiration, air in the conducting zone (part of the previous breath out) and the first part of the new breath reaches the lung tissue for gas exchange. The last part of the new breath stays within the conducting zone (and will be breathed back out again). Although dead space volume can be called wasted breathing, it is normal for everyone to have some. It extends from the nose and mouth to the terminal bronchioles. However, some lung diseases will increase the dead space volume.

Airway generations 20 to 28 are called the **respiratory zone** because there is some gas exchange through them. These airways are the smallest and lie within the lung tissue so that some oxygen and carbon dioxide can diffuse through them and into blood. The **alveolar sacs** and **alveoli** are the final generation of the airways. This is where most gas is exchanged between the lungs and the blood, as discussed in more detail later.

The trachea is the main airway and the largest (Figure 1-5). In an adult it is about 1.5 to 2.5 **centimeters (cm)** in diameter (between a dime and a quarter size). The trachea starts at the lower end of the larynx and ends in about the

Table 1-1 Major structures and corresponding generations of the tracheobronchial tree

	Structures of the Lungs	Generations*	
Conducting Zone	Trachea	0	Cartilaginous airways
	Main stem bronchi	1	
	Lobar bronchi	2	
	Segmental bronchi	3	
	Subsegmental bronchi	4–9	
	Bronchioles	10–15	Noncartilaginous airways
	Terminal bronchioles	16–19	
Respiratory Zone	Respiratory bronchioles[†]	20–23	Sites of gas exchange
	Alveolar ducts[†]	24–27	
	Alveolar sacs[†]	28	

*NOTE: The precise number of generations between the subsegmental bronchi and the alveolar sacs is not known.

[†]These structures collectively are referred to as a primary lobule or lung parenchyma; they are also called terminal respiratory units and functional units.

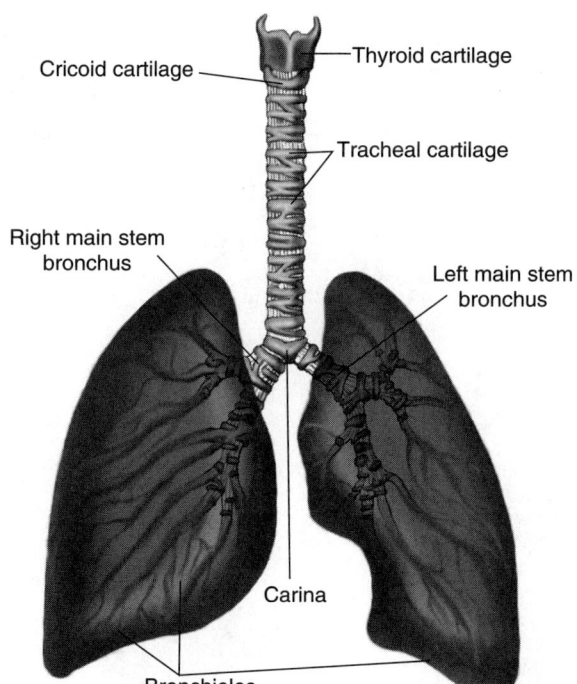

- **carina:** *the keel-shaped structure that projects from the lowest tracheal cartilage at the point where the trachea splits into the left and right mainstem bronchi*
- **left or right mainstem bronchus:** *the large airway that branches from the trachea and leads into a lung. (Plural, bronchi).*
- **lobe:** *a separate portion of any organ, such as the lobes of the lungs, brain, or liver*

Figure 1-5 Overall view of the tracheobronchial tree and lungs, as seen from the front

middle of the sternum (breastbone). At this level it splits into two at a place called the **carina.** These two branches are called the **left mainstem bronchus** and **right mainstem bronchus.** They enter the left and right lungs respectively. There is less of an angle to the right mainstem bronchus than the left. The right and left mainstem bronchi split into lobar bronchi. The right lung has an upper, middle, and lower **lobe.** The left lung has an upper and a lower lobe. The third generation of airways is the segmental bronchi, which lead to the numerous **segments** of the five lobes. There are 10 segments in the right lung and 8 segments in the left lung. There are between four and nine generations of subsegmental bronchi. These are the last generations of bronchi to have any cartilage to support their shape. These subsegmental bronchi have a diameter of about 1 to 4 **millimeters (mm)**—about the thickness of a pencil lead.

The next 10 generations of conducting zone airways are called *noncartilaginous airways,* because they have no cartilage to support their shape. The airway tissues and surrounding spiral/smooth muscles provide the only support (Figure 1-6). Airway generations 10 to 15 are called **bronchioles.** They are less than 1 mm in diameter. The last four generations of airways are called the **terminal bronchioles.** They are about 0.5 mm in diameter. They are the last airway generations of the conducting zone; no gas is exchanged through them. These noncartilaginous airways and the next generations of airways in the respiratory zone are frequently the site of respiratory disease. This is because of their lack of cartilage support. The respiratory zone airways are discussed later, with the lungs, because oxygen and carbon dioxide are exchanged through them.

The Mucociliary Escalator

The lungs' main protection against inhaled dust, pollen, and most **bacteria** is the inner lining of the airways (Figures 1-6 and 1-7). This inner lining is commonly called the **mucociliary escalator** because a layer of **mucus** is pushed by hair-like **cilia** from the terminal bronchioles to the top of the trachea. From there the mucus is swallowed or coughed out. The majority of mucus is excreted from the **submucosal glands** (also called bronchial glands or mucus glands).

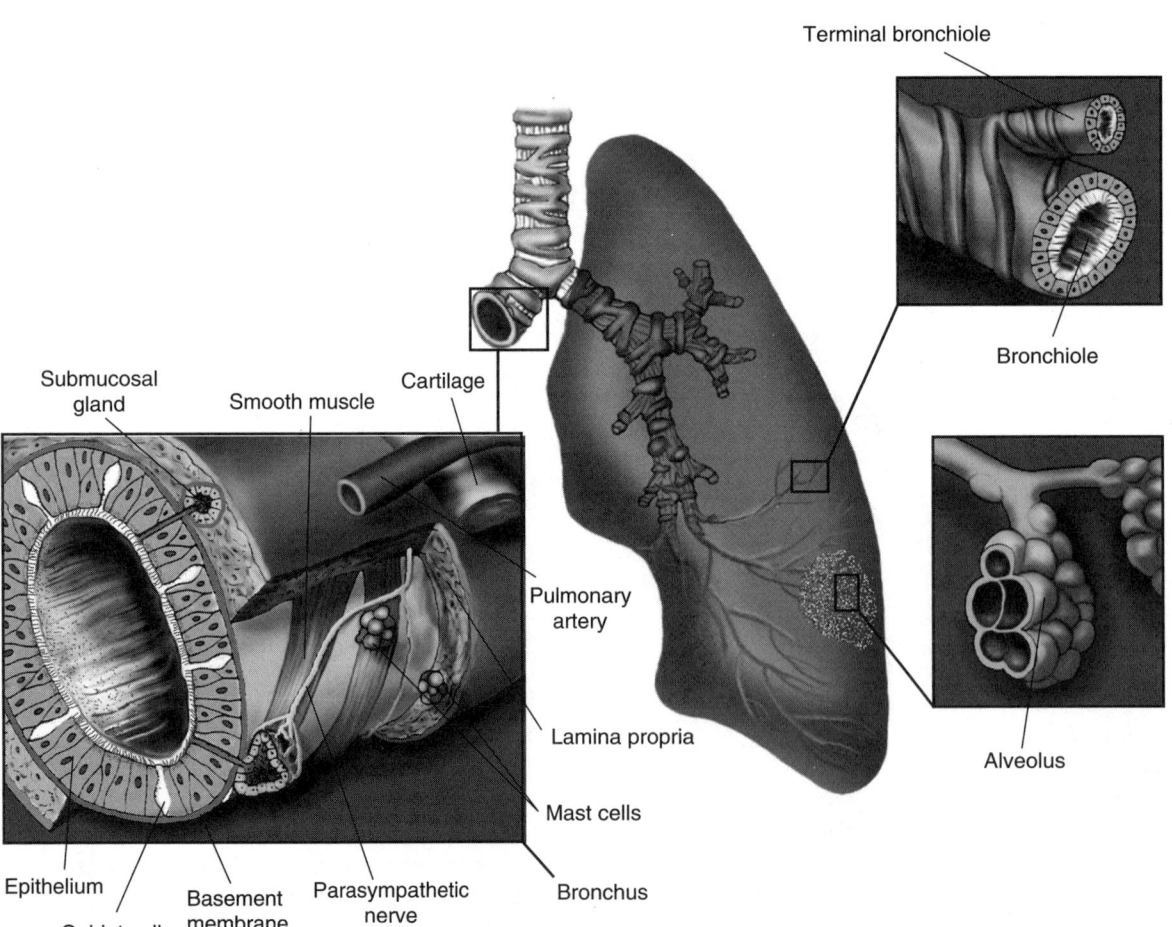

Figure 1-6   Subsections of the airways and lungs showing magnified views of a bronchus, bronchiole, and alveolar sac with alveolus

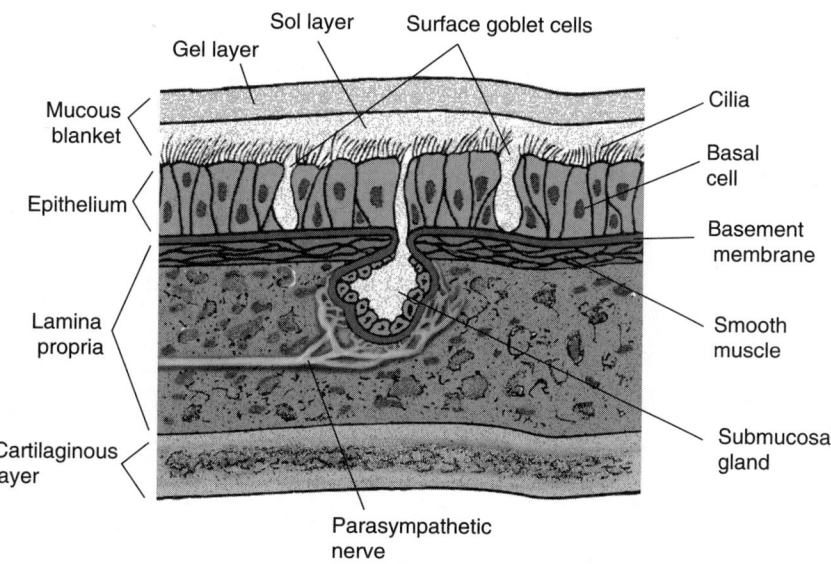

Figure 1-7   Magnified view of the structures of the wall of the mucociliary escalator and tracheobronchial tree

---

■ **mucociliary escalator:** *the mucus-clearing system of the respiratory passages; consists of the mucus layer and the cilia that push mucus out of the lungs*

■ **mucus:** *the viscous, slippery secretions of mucous membranes and glands, containing mucin, white blood cells, water, inorganic salts, and old cells. In the airway it separates into two layers. The inner layer (in contact with the tissues), called the* sol *layer, is mainly water. The outer layer (in contact with the air), called the* gel *layer, is sticky and traps inhaled dust and other particles*

■ **cilia:** *small, hairlike structures on the outer surfaces of some bronchial wall cells that aid in mucus clearance by producing motion in the liquid*

■ **submucosal glands:** *mucus-secreting glands found beneath the surface layer of cells of the airways; also called* bronchial glands *or* mucus glands

■ **autonomic nervous system:** *the part of the nervous system that regulates involuntary vital function, including the activity of glands, smooth muscles, and the activity of cardiac muscle. It has two divisions: the sympathetic nervous system accelerates heart rate, dilates the airways, constricts blood vessels, and raises blood pressure; the para-sympathetic nervous system slows heart rate, constricts the airways, increases intestinal movement, and relaxes sphincter muscles*

■ **surface goblet cell:** *one of the specialized mucus-secreting cells found in the lining of the respiratory tract, stomach, and intestine*

■ **parenchyma:** *the tissue of an organ, as distinguished from supporting or connective tissue; the part of the lung where gases are exchanged*

They normally release about 100 milliliters (mL) of mucus per day in an adult. More is released if an infection is present or inhaled dusts and pollens stimulate the gland's attached parasympathetic nervous system nerves. Parasympathetic nerves are part of the **autonomic nervous system.** Some mucus is also released from **surface goblet cells** (also called *goblet cells*). They also react to inhaled irritants. The submucosal glands and surface goblet cells are found from the trachea to the terminal bronchioles. The combined secretions from these two sources separate into two layers sometimes called the *mucus blanket.* The innermost layer, which is mostly water, is called the *sol layer.* The outermost layer is called the *gel layer.* It has less water, is sticky, and traps the inhaled dust, bacteria, and other foreign particles. The mucus layer is pushed out of the lungs by the action of the cilia. The cilia are small hair-like structures that originate in special cells within the epithelium lining the airway. They rapidly beat or wave in a coordinated manner and are found from the larynx to the level of the respiratory bronchioles. Normally, ciliary action pushes the mucus toward the trachea and larynx at a rate of about 20 mm per minute. Infection of the airways, tobacco smoke, and some harmful gases can slow down or stop ciliary movement.

The Lungs

The lungs are the structures where oxygen and carbon dioxide are exchanged. As mentioned earlier, the two lungs are divided into lobes and then segments (Figure 1-8). The right lung is slightly larger than the left and contains three lobes. The upper lobe has three segments; the middle lobe has two segments; the lower lobe has five segments. The left lung is slightly smaller than the right and is shaped to make room for the heart. The left lung has an upper lobe with two divisions; each division has two segments. The upper division has two combined segments. The lower segment, called the *lingula,* is part of the upper lobe but corresponds to the middle lobe of the right lung. The lower lobe of the left lung has four segments; two are combined. Remember, each lobe has its own lobar bronchus and each segment has its own segmental bronchus. Additionally, each segment has its own artery, vein, and vessels of the lymphatic system. (These are discussed later.)

The lung **parenchyma** is the actual gas exchange area of the pulmonary system. The parenchyma of each lung is made up of about 150,000 gas exchange

Right lung		Left lung	
Upper lobe		Upper lobe	
Apical	1	Upper division	
Posterior	2	Apical/Posterior	1 & 2
Anterior	3	Anterior	3
Middle lobe		Lower division (lingular)	
Lateral	4	Superior lingula	4
Medial	5	Inferior lingula	5
Lower lobe		Lower lobe	
Superior	6	Superior	6
Medial basal	7	Anterior medial	7 & 8
Anterior basal	8	Lateral basal	9
Lateral basal	9	Posterior basal	10
Posterior basal	10		

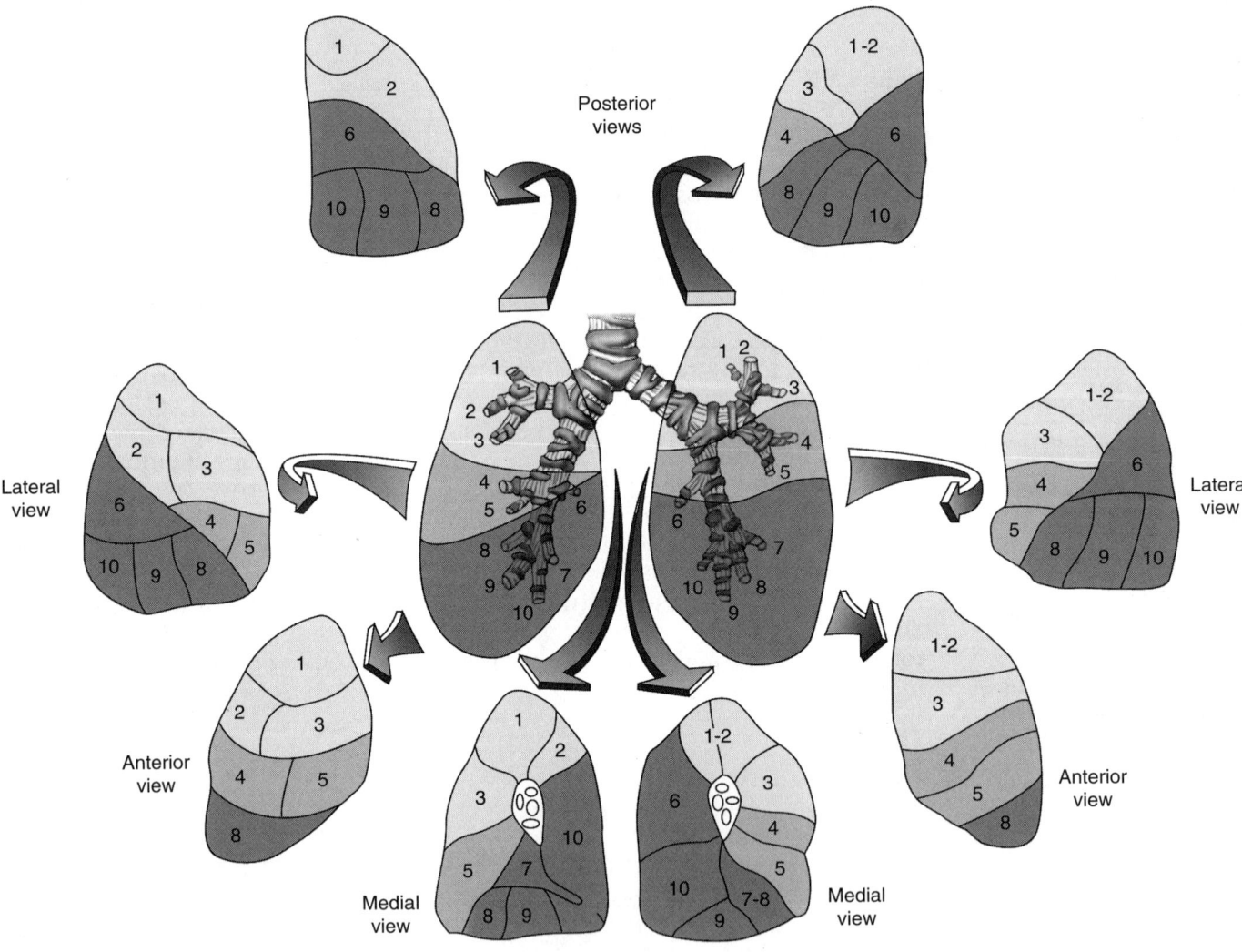

Figure 1-8   The segments of the lungs. The basic segments of the right and left lung are the same. However, many believe that because several segments of the left lung are combined, there are only eight segments instead of ten as in the right lung.

■ acinus: *a subdivision of the lung consisting of the tissue distal to the terminal bronchiole; also called* primary lobule *or* alveolus

■ respiratory bronchiole: *a small division of the respiratory system extending from the terminal bronchiole to the alveolar ducts. Gases directly diffuse through alveoli in its wall as well as flowing through its lumen between alveoli ducts and the terminal airway*

■ alveolar duct: *any of the air passages in the lung that branch out from the respiratory bronchioles. From the ducts arise the alveolar sacs*

■ capillary: *one of the tiny blood vessels (about 0.008 mm in diameter) joining arterioles and venules. Gases and other substances diffuse through their walls*

■ alveolus: *a single, small, saclike structure in the lung where gas exchange takes place*

■ pores of Kohn: *small openings between the cells making up the walls of alveoli. These openings allow gases to diffuse between adjacent alveoli in different alveolar sacs*

■ alveolar-capillary membrane: *a lung tissue structure that is about 0.001 mm thick, through which diffusion of oxygen and carbon dioxide molecules occurs during the respiration process. It consists of an alveolar cell separated from a capillary cell by an interstitial space and is essentially a fluid barrier*

■ type I cell: *a thin-walled cell that makes up about 95% of the alveolar surface area; the cell through which gases exchange with the adjoining capillaries*

units. Each is called an **acinus** or primary lobule and is composed of the **respiratory bronchioles, alveolar ducts,** alveolar sacs, and alveoli that come from a single terminal bronchiole. This is the respiratory zone as shown in Table 1-1. Because of the closeness of the pulmonary **capillaries** and the thinness of the tissues, oxygen and carbon dioxide (and other gases) can diffuse back and forth. The respiratory bronchioles have some alveoli budding from them. The alveolar ducts are made up of alveoli that are supported by thin walls containing smooth muscle fibers. The alveolar ducts end in alveolar sacs. They look like clusters of grapes and are made up of about 15 to 20 alveoli. The alveoli fit edge to edge. Each individual **alveolus** is 0.2 mm in diameter and only the thickness of the alveolar cell (Figures 1-6 and 1-9). There are occasional small openings between adjoining alveolar sacs that are called **pores of Kohn.** The pores of Kohn allow gases to move between the neighboring alveolar sacs. It is estimated that an adult has a total of 300 million alveoli with a surface area of about 70 square meters. This is about the size of a tennis court! The pulmonary capillaries cover 85% to 95% of the surface of the alveoli. The combination of the alveoli and pulmonary capillaries is called the **alveolar-capillary membrane.** This membrane is the place where most of the respiratory gases are exchanged. Only small amounts of oxygen and carbon dioxide are exchanged in the respiratory bronchioles and alveolar ducts.

The alveoli are made up of two different types of cells. Most of the surface area is made up by the thin-walled **type I cell.** This is the cell through which gases

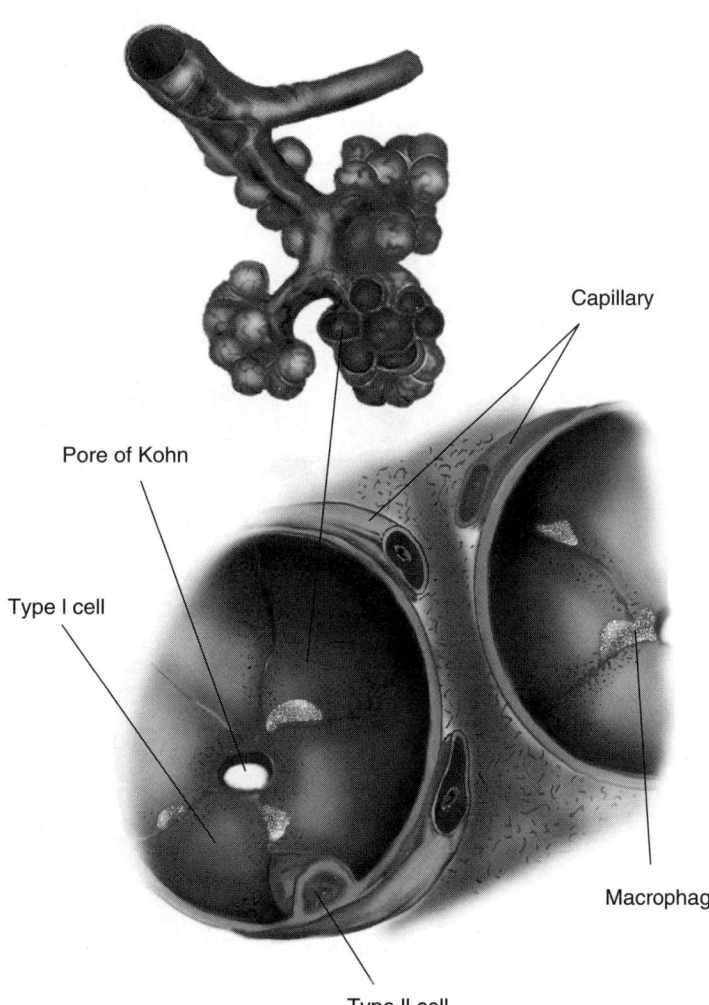

Figure 1-9
Magnified view of the alveolar sac and alveolar-capillary membrane, showing structures

■ *type II cell: a thick, cuboidal cell that makes up about 5% of the alveolar surface area; the cell that makes the surface-tension-reducing substance surfactant*

■ *surfactant: certain lipoproteins that reduce the surface tension of pulmonary liquids, allowing the alveoli of the lungs to stay open for gas exchange*

■ *surface tension: the tendency of a liquid to minimize the area of its surface by contracting; this property affects the size of the alveoli by causing them to become smaller or collapse*

■ *alveolar macrophages: defense cells within the lungs that act by engulfing and digesting foreign substances, such as bacteria, that may be inhaled into the alveoli*

■ *thorax: the cage of bone and cartilage containing the heart and lungs and covering part of the abdominal organs. It is formed ventrally by the sternum and costal cartilages and dorsally by the 12 thoracic vertebrae and dorsal parts of the 12 ribs on each side*

■ *inspiration (inhalation): the act of drawing air into the lungs to exchange oxygen for carbon dioxide*

diffuse. The second is called the **type II cell.** It is thicker and serves the purpose of making a vital substance called **surfactant.** Surfactant is chemically related to fat. It acts like soap to lower the **surface tension** of the water layer that lines the inside of each alveolus. Without surfactant, the surface tension within the alveoli would cause them to collapse. Obviously, collapsed alveoli cannot contain air and oxygen and carbon dioxide cannot diffuse through them.

A third cell is found within the alveoli but is not part of the alveolar structure. These cells are called **alveolar macrophages** (Figure 1-9). They are specialized, mobile cells of the immune system and are the last line of defense of the lung. Macrophages are able to move about and ingest and kill most bacteria and other invading pathogens. However, they cannot effectively remove other substances such as silica dust or asbestos fibers.

There is one other pulmonary structure of special interest. This is the system of lymphatic vessels (Figure 1-10). They have the job of removing any excess fluid from around the alveoli. Commonly some plasma-type fluid leaks out of the pulmonary capillaries. If the fluid is not removed, it will leak into the alveoli. The lymphatic vessels remove this excess fluid and eventually drain it back into the venous system.

Thorax and Abdomen

The **thorax** is usually called the chest. The thorax protects the heart, lungs, and related structures from injury and also is a vital part of the pulmonary system.

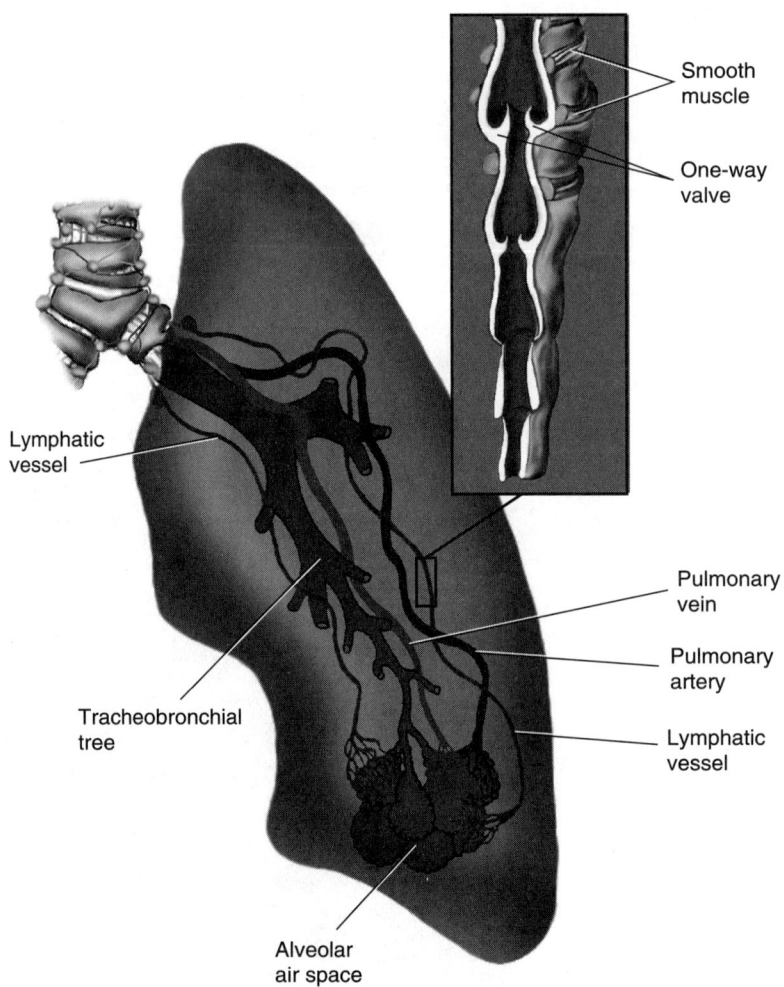

Smooth muscle

One-way valve

Lymphatic vessel

Pulmonary vein

Pulmonary artery

Lymphatic vessel

Tracheobronchial tree

Alveolar air space

Figure 1-10   Magnified view of a lymphatic vessel and related structures

■ *expiration (exhalation):* breathing out, normally a passive process, depending on the elastic qualities of lung tissue and the thorax

■ *mediastinum:* a portion of the thoracic cavity in the middle of the thorax between the pleural sacs containing the two lungs

■ *hilum:* a depression or pit in each lung where the mainstem bronchus, vessels, and nerves enter

■ *fetus:* the human being in utero from the eighth week after fertilization until birth

■ *pericardium:* a fibroserous sac that surrounds the heart and great vessels. Pericardial fluid lies between the two layers and acts as a lubricant so that the heart easily moves during contraction. Also known as the pericardial sac

■ *pleura:* a delicate serous membrane enclosing each lung. The pleura divides into the visceral pleura, which covers the lung, and the parietal pleura, which lines the chest wall and covers the diaphragm and the structures in the mediastinum

The so-called thoracic cage or rib cage is made up of the spine in back, the twelve ribs that attach to the spine and wrap around the sides, and the sternum (breast bone) that joins most of the ribs together in front (Figure 1-11). Only the first seven ribs, counting from the top, directly attach to the sternum by cartilage. The next three ribs are indirectly attached to the sternum by cartilage. The bottom two ribs are not attached to the sternum. Because of this they are called the *floating ribs.* The spaces between the ribs (intercostal spaces) are filled by blood vessels, nerves, and the internal and external intercostal muscles. Besides protecting the lungs and heart, the rib cage helps in breathing. When the muscles of **inspiration (inhalation)** contract, the lower ribs move outward to the front and sides. This increases the volume of the lungs. As a result, the air pressure drops in the lungs and fresh air is pulled into them. During vigorous exercise, the upper ribs are also lifted outward so that even more air can be brought into the lungs. At the end of a breath, the muscles relax and the ribs spring back to their resting place. This causes the lungs to become smaller and air to be pushed out for an **expiration (exhalation).**

The area between the lungs is called the **mediastinum.** The **hilum** of each lung is within it. Additionally, the heart, large blood vessels, esophagus, and trachea are contained within the mediastinum (Figure 1-12).

As the heart and lungs develop in the **fetus,** they grow into their own flexible, double-layered membranes that enclose them. The heart grows into the double layered **pericardium.** Each lung is contained within a double-layered membrane called the **pleura.** The inner membrane is called the *visceral pleura* and lies over each lung. The outer membrane is called the *parietal pleura* and covers the inside of the rib cage, diaphragm, and mediastinal structures. A small amount of pleural fluid is contained within the pleural cavity. This fluid lubricates the pleural surfaces so that ribs and lungs easily move over each other during breathing.

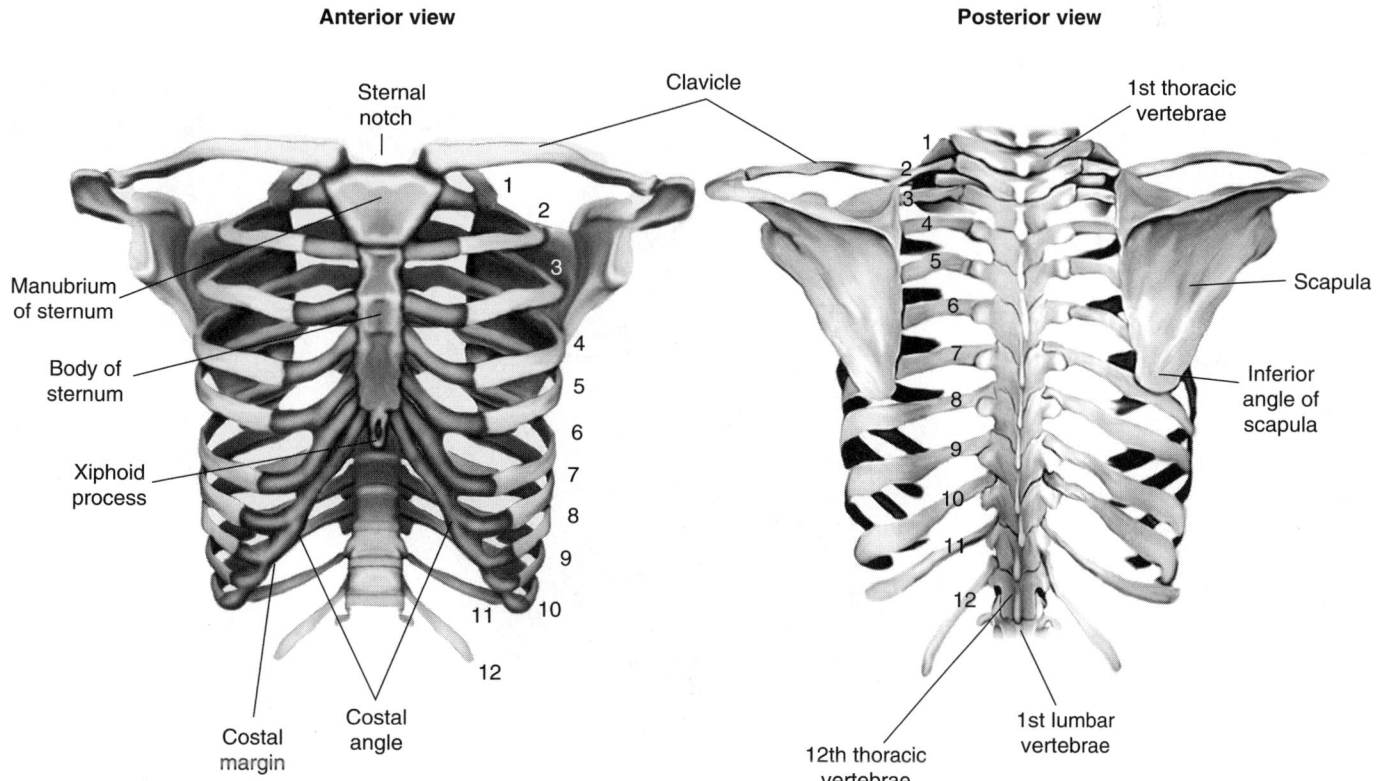

Figure 1-11   The thoracic cage/rib cage, showing the ribs, sternum, vertebrae, and associated bones

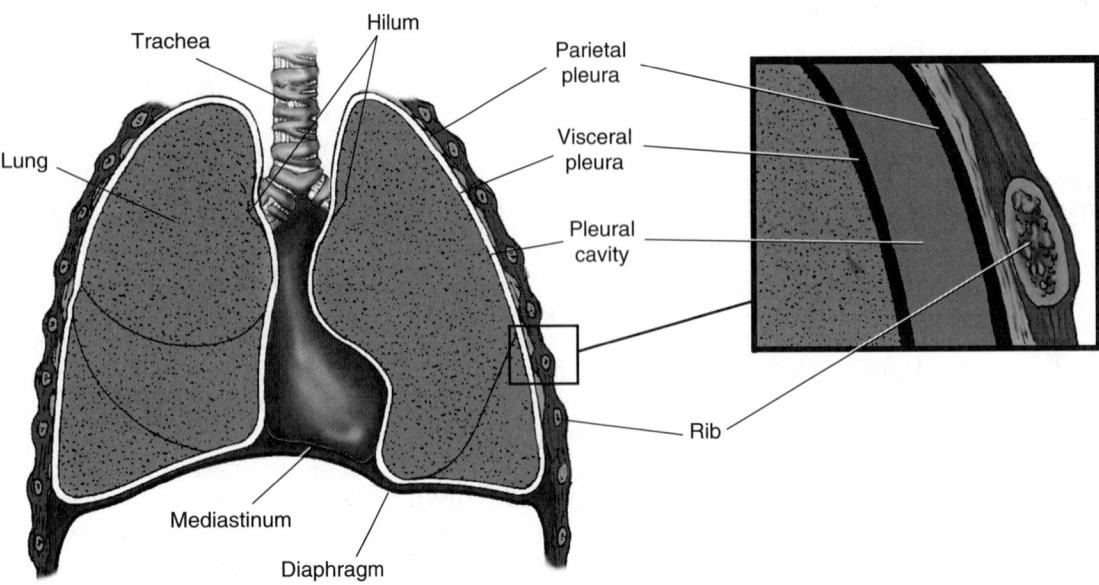

Figure 1-12   Major structures around the lungs, the mediastinum, and a magnified view of the pleural cavity

■ **diaphragm:** *a dome-shaped musculofibrous partition that separates the thoracic and abdominal cavities. It is the main muscle of breathing. During inspiration it moves down and increases the volume of the thoracic cavity; during expiration it moves up, decreasing the volume*

■ **hemidiaphragm:** *either the left or right functional half of the diaphragm. Although the structure is a single anatomic unit, it is divided by the union of its central tendon and the pericardium into separate leaves, each with its own nerve supply. Each hemidiaphragm can function independently of the other*

■ **inferior vena cava:** *the large vein that returns unoxygenated blood to the heart from parts of the body below the diaphragm*

■ **aorta:** *the main trunk of the systemic arterial circulation, comprising four parts: the ascending aorta, the arch of the aorta, the thoracic portion of the descending aorta, and the abdominal portion of the descending aorta*

The **diaphragm** is a large, flat sheet of muscle that separates the thoracic organs from the abdominal organs (Figure 1-13). Actually, the diaphragm is made up of two different but joined muscles. They are the right and left **hemidiaphragms.** However, for the sake of simplicity, these two muscles are often referred to simply as the diaphragm. It is the main muscle of breathing. Below the diaphragm lie the abdominal organs. The liver is immediately below the right hemidiaphragm. The stomach is below the left hemidiaphragm. The **inferior vena cava, aorta,** and esophagus pass through natural openings in the diaphragm.

Muscles of Breathing

The diaphragm is the main muscle used during quiet breathing. As mentioned earlier, it is really two muscles. The right and left hemidiaphragms are joined

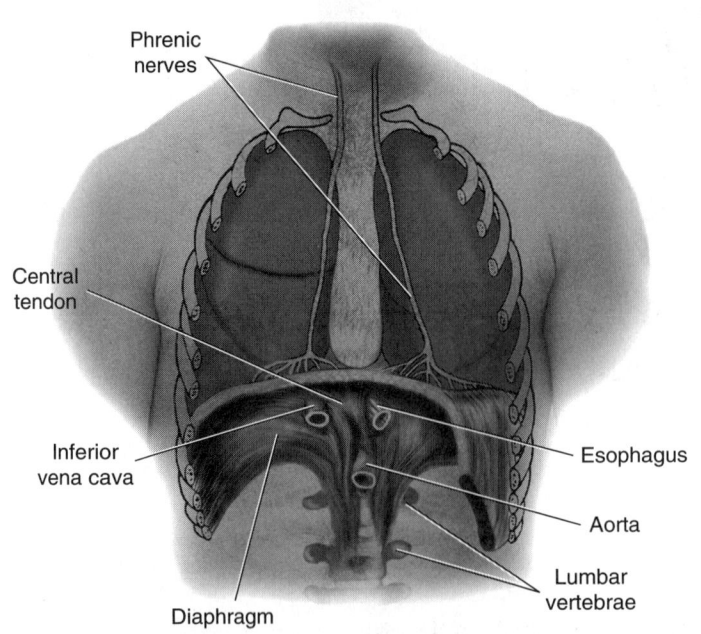

Figure 1-13 The diaphragm, phrenic nerves, and related structures

together in the middle by a central tendon. Normally the two hemidiaphragms work together in a coordinated effort. It is common practice to refer to the diaphragm as a single muscle, so we will do so here also. When the diaphragm contracts, it pulls down. This forces the lower ribs outward to the front and sides and the abdominal contents down and out. The pulling down of the diaphragm results in the lungs being pulled down. This causes a drop in pressure within the lungs, so outside air is pulled in to give a breath.

During vigorous exercise, or in patients with lung disease, additional muscles are often used to help with inspiration. These are the accessory muscles of inspiration:

■ External intercostal muscles, found between the ribs (Figure 1-14)
■ Scalene muscles, found on both sides of the neck
■ Sternocleidomastoid muscles, also found on both sides of the neck
■ Trapezius muscles, found on both sides of the upper back and neck
■ Pectoralis major muscles, found on both sides of the upper front of the chest

The accessory muscles of inspiration work together to pull the upper ribs up and out. If you see a patient using these accessory muscles, it is a sign of respiratory distress. Contact the nurse, physician, or **respiratory care practitioner (RCP)** for assistance.

Normally, resting expiration is passive. As mentioned earlier, when the inspiratory muscles relax, the ribs recoil back to their resting position. Additionally, the relaxed diaphragm rises up and the abdominal contents move back into their resting position. The lungs are pushed up into the thorax and made smaller. The air pressure rises within the shrinking lungs and the air is pushed out, causing exhalation.

Hint: *Check this by putting your hands over your lower ribs and your abdomen as you breathe.*

Hint: *Check this by putting your hands over your upper chest and neck as you take in and hold a full breath.*

■ *respiratory care practitioner (RCP): the general term used to describe an allied health professional who specializes in scientific knowledge and theory of clinical problems of respiratory care. Duties include collecting and evaluating patient information to determine an appropriate care plan, selecting and assembling equipment, conducting therapeutic procedures, and modifying prescribed care plans to achieve one or more specific objectives. Practitioners hold either the Certified Respiratory Therapy Technician (CRTT) or Registered Respiratory Therapist (RRT) credential*

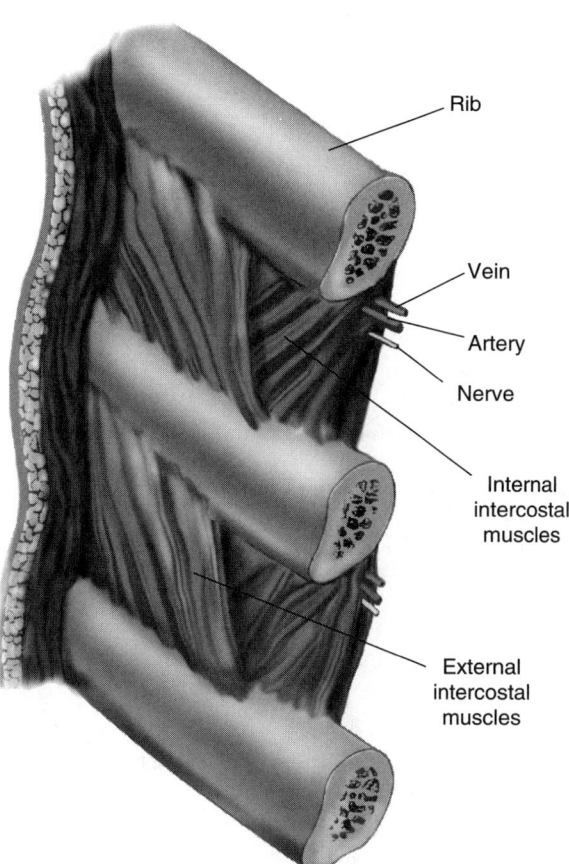

Rib

Vein

Artery

Nerve

Internal intercostal muscles

External intercostal muscles

Figure 1-14 The intercostal space, showing accessory muscles of inspiration and expiration

During vigorous exercise, or in patients with lung disease, additional muscles are used to speed up exhalation. These are the accessory muscles of exhalation:

- Internal intercostal muscles, found between the ribs (Figure 1-14)
- Rectus abdominis muscles, found in the front of the abdominal wall
- External abdominal oblique (obliquus externus abdominis) muscles, found on both sides of the lower chest and upper abdominal wall
- Internal abdominal oblique (obliquus internus abdominis) muscles, found on both sides of the lower chest and abdominal wall
- Transversus abdominis muscles, found on both sides of the lower chest and abdominal wall

The combined effect of these sets of muscles is to pull the ribs down and in and to pull the abdominal contents in. The total effect of using these muscles is to rapidly force most of the air out of the lungs. This allows a person to inhale again more quickly, thus increasing the respiratory rate.

■■■ CONTROL OF BREATHING

The muscles of respiration would be useless if they did not get the proper commands from the right nerves at the right time. The breathing that most people take for granted all of their lives is the result of a series of steps of nervous system input to the brain and output from the brain. If the nervous system is damaged, the ability to breathe is altered or stopped altogether.

Respiratory Center of the Brain

An area of the brain called the **medulla oblongata** is the primary respiratory center. The secondary respiratory center of the brain is located in the **pons** (Figure 1-15). Both areas are located between the base of the brain and the spinal cord. Several sites within the medulla and pons influence inspiration and expiration:

- Dorsal respiratory group (DRG)—primary site for inspiratory signals to the diaphragm and other inspiratory muscles
- Ventral respiratory group (VRG)—during heavy exercise, sends signals to inspiratory and expiratory muscle groups
- Apneustic center (APC)—secondary site of inspiratory signals to the DRG and VRG

Hint: *Check this by placing your hands over your lower ribs and abdomen while blowing up a balloon or performing the Valsalva maneuver.*

■ *medulla oblongata: the most vital part of the entire brain, continuing as the bulbous portion of the spinal cord just above the foramen magnum and separated from the pons by a horizontal groove. The medulla contains the cardiac, the vasomotor, and the respiratory centers of the brain*

■ *pons: a bulge on the ventral surface of the brainstem, between the medulla oblongata and the cerebral peduncles*

■ *hydrogen ion (H+): a positively charged hydrogen atom nucleus. Hydrogen is the simplest and lightest of the elements and is colorless, odorless, and highly flammable. As a component of water, hydrogen is crucial in the metabolic interaction of acids, bases, and salts within the body and in the fluid balance necessary for the body to survive*

■ *hypoxemia: an abnormal deficiency of oxygen in the arterial blood. Symptoms of acute hypoxemia are restlessness, stupor, coma, abnormal breathing pattern, apnea (no breathing), increased and then decreased cardiac output and blood pressure, ventricular fibrillation, and/or asystole. Death can result*

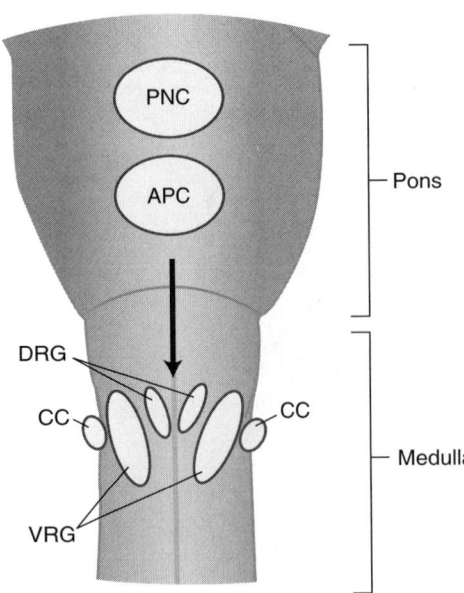

Figure 1-15 The respiratory center of the brain. The medulla oblongata contains the dorsal respiratory group (DRG), ventral respiratory group (VRG), and central chemoreceptors (CC). The pons contains the pneumotaxic center (PNC) and the apneustic center (APC). The main part of the brain is located above the pons and the spinal cord is located below the medulla.

- Pneumotaxic center (PNC)—secondary site of inspiratory signals leading to rapid, shallow breathing
- Central chemoreceptors (CC)—influence all of the other nerve centers

The central chemoreceptors and the other nerve sites are stimulated by **hydrogen ions (H$^+$).** Hydrogen ions are mainly released from a chemical reaction between carbon dioxide and water that takes place in the fluid surrounding the brain. Remember from the earlier discussion that carbon dioxide (CO_2) is a waste product of metabolism. Our lungs remove it when we exhale. The brain, in effect, monitors how much carbon dioxide is in the body and directs the lungs to breathe to blow it off. Carbon dioxide is the primary driving force behind our need to breathe. Many people are under the impression that we breathe to take in oxygen, but it really is to get rid of CO_2!

Hypoxic Drive to Breathe

Most patients with heart or lung disease will have a low level of oxygen in their blood **(hypoxemia).** This results in a low level of oxygen in the cells of the body; such a patient is said to be **hypoxic.** This dangerous situation is the second driving force behind the need to breathe. If the brain were injured or not responding normally to the level of carbon dioxide, we would not breathe unless there were another stimulus. Having a low oxygen level is, in effect, a backup system that keeps us breathing if the brain is not responding normally to carbon dioxide. The brain is less sensitive to CO_2 when a person has been given an overdose of sedative or pain-relieving drugs, or when a person has severe lung disease and cannot blow off enough carbon dioxide.

There are special oxygen-sensitive cells found in **carotid bodies** in the **carotid arteries** and **aortic bodies** in the aorta (Figure 1-16). When a person

- **hypoxic:** having inadequate oxygen at the cellular level; a condition that can result in death
- **carotid body:** a small structure containing neural tissue at the bifurcation of the carotid arteries; monitors the oxygen content of the blood and assists in regulating breathing
- **carotid arteries:** two main arteries that branch off the aorta and supply blood to the head
- **aortic bodies:** small structures containing neural tissue located in the aorta; they monitor the oxygen content of the blood and assist in regulating breathing

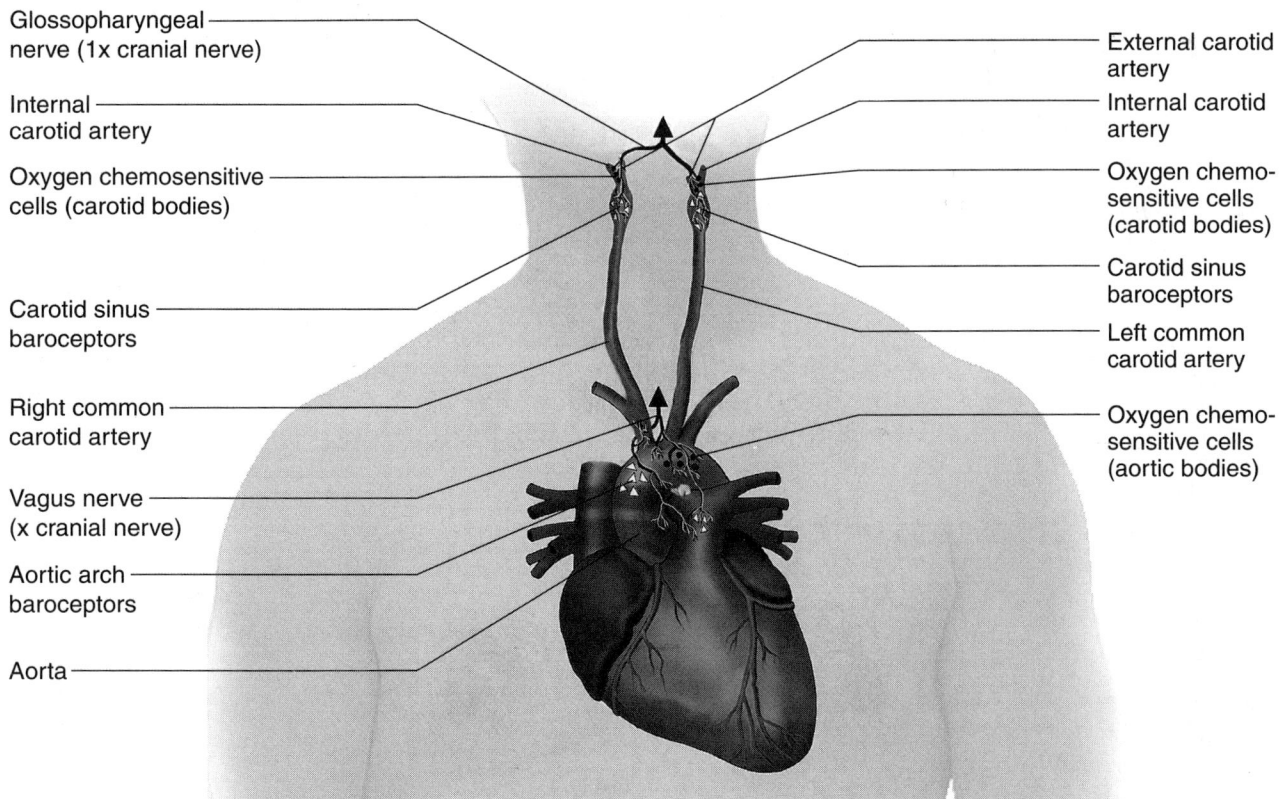

Glossopharyngeal nerve (1x cranial nerve)

Internal carotid artery

Oxygen chemosensitive cells (carotid bodies)

Carotid sinus baroceptors

Right common carotid artery

Vagus nerve (x cranial nerve)

Aortic arch baroceptors

Aorta

External carotid artery

Internal carotid artery

Oxygen chemo-sensitive cells (carotid bodies)

Carotid sinus baroceptors

Left common carotid artery

Oxygen chemo-sensitive cells (aortic bodies)

Figure 1-16 Locations of the carotid and aortic bodies (the peripheral chemoreceptors). Breathing is stimulated when they sense hypoxemia. The baroreceptors sense blood pressure.

Note: *The preceding information on carbon dioxide and oxygen levels and stimulation of breathing applies to most patients. There are certain patients with chronic lung disease who are not given enough extra oxygen to bring their blood oxygen level back to normal. To completely correct the hypoxemia of these chronic lung disease patients would blunt their drive to breathe. If you are ever in doubt about a patient's breathing efforts or receiving extra oxygen, contact the physician, nurse, or respiratory care practitioner.*

has hypoxemia, these oxygen-sensitive bodies are stimulated and send signals to the respiratory center of the brain. The person is then stimulated to breathe and take in more oxygen. Carbon dioxide will now also be blown off.

Because hypoxemia is a very dangerous condition, it is usually treated by giving the patient extra oxygen to breathe. Methods of giving extra oxygen are discussed in Chapter 3. However, it is important to know that not all patients are treated the same. There are times when too much oxygen can be dangerous.

Cough Reflex and Sneeze Reflex

Who has not inhaled some dust and sneezed, or swallowed some food "down the wrong pipe" and coughed? Probably everyone has at least once. These two reactions help to keep the airways clear of foreign matter. In the case of the cough reflex, it might be lifesaving. Food or drink in the airways will plug them and prevent air movement. Additionally, food that stays in the airway can lead to an infection. The cough reflex is started when foreign matter irritates the larynx, trachea, carina, or bronchi. Additionally, if irritating chemicals in the air reach the terminal bronchioles or alveoli, a cough is stimulated. Any of these events trigger nerves in the airways, which send a signal to the brain. The following events then take place:

1. A deep breath is taken.
2. The epiglottis and vocal cords close.
3. The abdominal muscles contract and force the diaphragm up, greatly increasing the pressure in the lungs.
4. The epiglottis and vocal cords suddenly open.
5. Air from the lungs is rapidly blown out through the mouth along with the food or other substance.

A sneeze is caused when something such as dust, powder, or pollen is inhaled into the nasal passages. The nerves in the nasal passages then send a signal to the brain. With one exception, the events in the cough reflex happen again. With the sneeze, at event 5 the uvula is depressed toward the tongue so that the air is blasted out through the nose instead of the mouth. This usually clears away the nasal irritant.

Voluntary Control of Breathing

Normally we do not think about the need to breathe. The preceding discussion covered how the body automatically regulates breathing. However, there are times when we can consciously either increase or decrease how often or how deeply we breathe. For example, taking a deep breath to swim under water, blowing up a balloon, or blowing out candles on a birthday cake demonstrate voluntary control of breathing. Most people can only hold their breath for about 30 seconds before feeling the need to breathe again. The buildup of carbon dioxide and the drop in oxygen are both powerful stimulators! After taking a few deep breaths to restore normal levels of both gases, the body will go back to breathing normally.

Hint: *Time how long you can hold your breath before feeling the need to breathe again.*

phrenic nerves: *a pair of nerves that arise from between the third and fifth cervical vertebrae. They extend through the thorax to provide innervation to the diaphragm. The right phrenic nerve stimulates the right hemidiaphragm and the left phrenic nerve stimulates the left hemidiaphragm*

Key Concept: *A patient with a known or suspected neck vertebral injury will always wear a neck brace until it has been proven that there is no injury to the spinal cord.*

Nerves to the Muscles of Breathing

The diaphragm is stimulated mainly by the **phrenic nerves** (Figure 1-13). Each hemidiaphragm has its own nerve. The phrenic nerves originate between the third and fifth cervical (neck) segments (vertebrae) of the spinal cord. The accessory muscles of ventilation are stimulated by nerves originating from the thoracic or lumbar vertebrae.

CIRCULATORY SYSTEM

The human circulatory system is made up of two major sections. The pulmonary section takes blood through the lungs to pick up oxygen and drop off carbon dioxide. The systemic section takes blood throughout the body to drop off oxygen and pick up carbon dioxide. Both sections must function individually and together to maintain good health.

The Heart as a Pump

The heart functions as a muscular pump to push blood throughout the body. Located behind the protecting sternum, a person's heart is about the size of his or her fist (Figures 1-16 and 1-17). When the heart muscle contracts, the blood is squeezed out to the arteries. The heart is a unique muscle that seemingly never tires out (unlike the muscles in your arms or legs) and it has the ability to trigger its own contractions. It is easiest to feel the heart's contraction (often called the heartbeat) by placing your hand over your chest to the left side of the sternum. This is called the **apical pulse** and is felt over the heart's left ventricle. The surge of blood through the arteries can be felt in a number of locations throughout the body (Figure 1-18).

The rate at which the heart beats varies with age and activity level. In general, a younger person's heart beats faster than an older person's. In any person, the resting heart beats more slowly than when the person is exercising. See

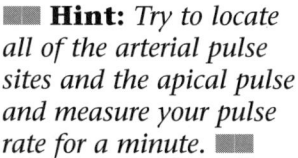 **Hint:** *Try to locate all of the arterial pulse sites and the apical pulse and measure your pulse rate for a minute.*

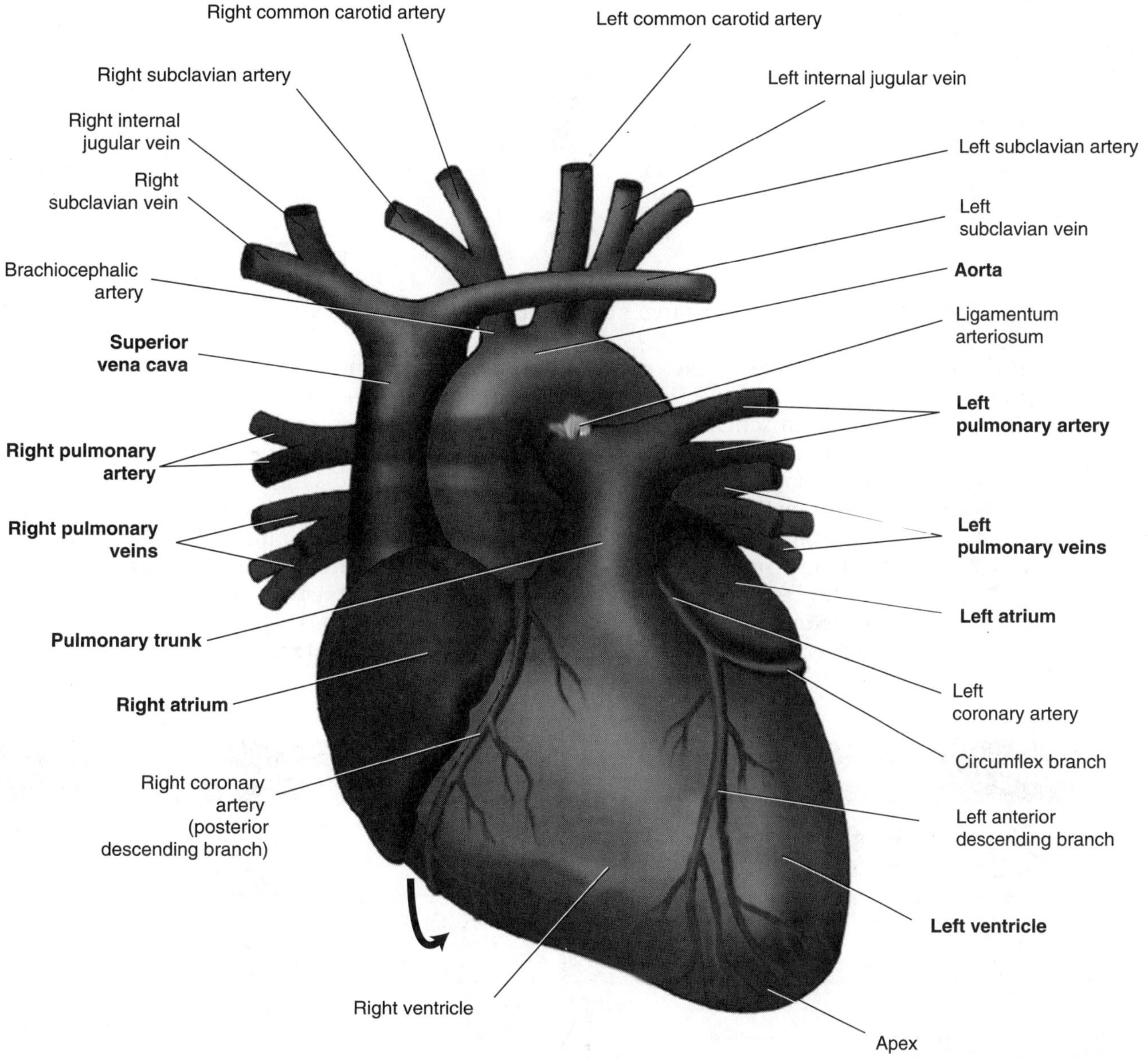

■ *apical pulse: the heart rate as felt over the chest or heard with a stethoscope placed over the chest wall adjacent to the cardiac apex*

Right common carotid artery

Left common carotid artery

Right subclavian artery

Left internal jugular vein

Right internal jugular vein

Left subclavian artery

Right subclavian vein

Left subclavian vein

Brachiocephalic artery

Aorta

Ligamentum arteriosum

Superior vena cava

Left pulmonary artery

Right pulmonary artery

Right pulmonary veins

Left pulmonary veins

Pulmonary trunk

Left atrium

Right atrium

Left coronary artery

Right coronary artery (posterior descending branch)

Circumflex branch

Left anterior descending branch

Left ventricle

Right ventricle

Apex

Figure 1-17 Anterior (front) view of the heart and associated vessels

■ *sinoatrial node (SA node):* a cluster of cells located in the right atrial wall of the heart, near the opening of the superior vena cava. It comprises a knot of modified heart muscle that generates impulses that travel swiftly throughout the muscle fibers of both atria, causing them to contract. Specialized pacemaker cells in this node have an intrinsic rhythm that is independent of any stimulation by nerve impulses from the brain and spinal cord. The SA node normally "fires" at a rhythmic rate of 70 to 75 beats per minute

■ *atrioventricular node (AV node):* an area of specialized cardiac muscle that receives the cardiac impulse from the sinoatrial node and conducts it to the bundle of His and then to the bundle branches and Purkinje fibers in the walls of the ventricles. The AV node is located in the septal wall of the right atrium

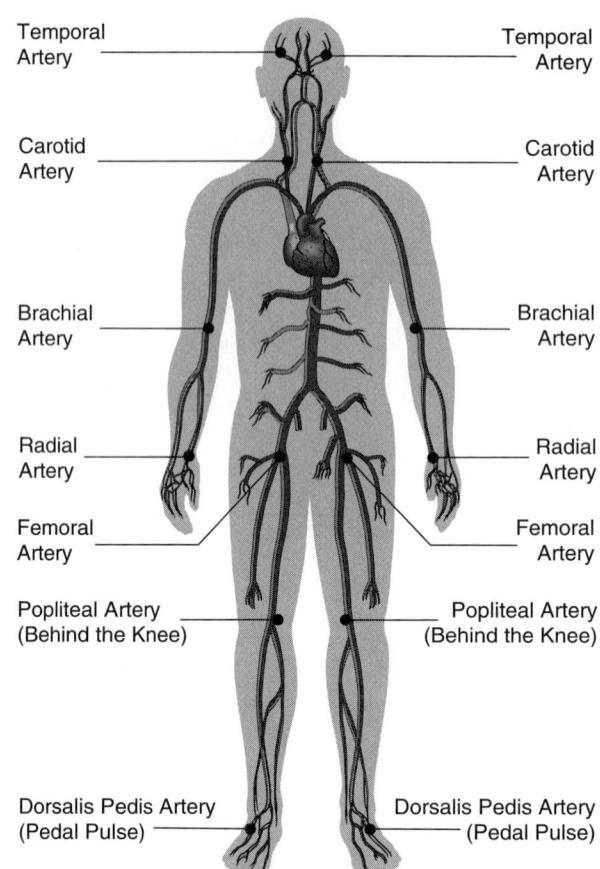

Figure 1-18 Main arteries and pulse points. The apical pulse can be felt by placing the hand over the chest to the left of the lower sternum.

■■ **Note:** *If you find a resting patient's heart rate to vary, or be slower or faster than expected, tell the nurse or RCP. If you cannot find a patient's heart rate, get help immediately! Begin cardiopulmonary resuscitation (CPR) if needed.* ■■

Table 1-2 for the ranges of resting heart rates for a young child, older child, and adult.

A number of factors work together to determine the best heart rate to pump enough blood to the body. Separate nerve centers in the medulla oblongata of the brain send nerve impulses to either speed up or slow down the heart rate. The body also makes chemicals to speed up the heart during emergencies. This is the so-called "fight or flight" response of the sympathetic nervous system. Additionally, the patient's physician may order medications to change the heart rate and strength of contraction. The heart has its own unique nerve conduction system. The parts of the conduction system are the **sinoatrial node (SA node), atrioventricular node (AV node), bundle of His,** left and right **bundle branches,** and **Purkinje fibers** (Figure 1-19). The normal pacemaker (starter of the heartbeat) is located in the right **atrium** in the SA node. The

Table 1-2 Normal ranges for resting respiratory rate, heart rate, and blood pressure			
	Respiratory Rate Per Minute	**Heart Rate Per Minute**	**Blood Pressure**
Adult	12–20	60–100	120/80 mm Hg (millimeters of mercury)
Older child	20–24	70–115	100/70 mm Hg
Young child	22–30	80–140	60/20 mm Hg

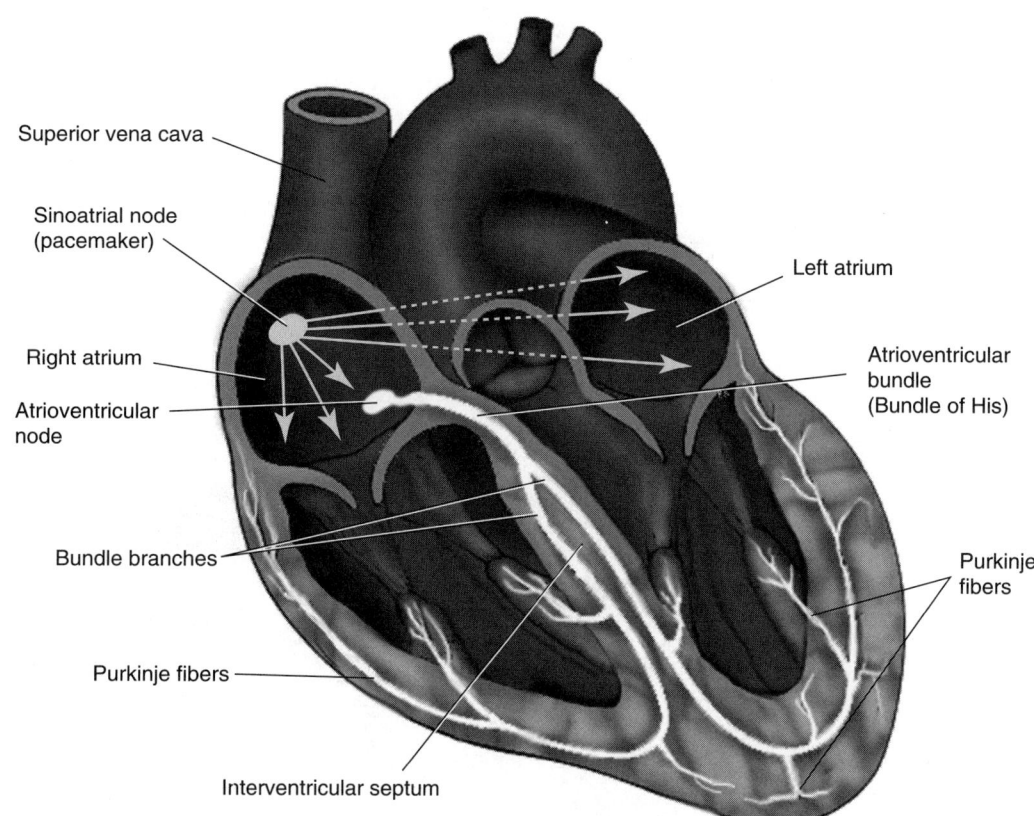

Figure 1-19   Electrical conduction system of the heart. The sinoatrial (SA) node is the normal pacemaker of the heart.

■ **bundle of His:** *a band of atypical cardiac muscle fibers with few contractile units. It arises from the distal portion of the AV node, where it divides into the bundle branches*

■ **bundle branches:** *a network of specialized conducting fibers that transmit electrical impulses throughout the right and left ventricles*

■ **Purkinje fibers:** *myocardial fibers that are a continuation of the bundle branches and extend into the muscle walls of the ventricles*

■ **atrium** *(plural,* **atria)***: one of the two upper chambers of the heart. The right atrium receives deoxygenated blood from the superior vena cava, inferior vena cava, and the coronary sinus. The left atrium receives oxygenated blood from the pulmonary veins. Blood is emptied into the ventricles from the atria*

■ **ventricles:** *the two larger chambers of the heart. The right ventricle is the lower chamber of the right side of the heart, which pumps venous blood through the pulmonary artery to the capillaries of the lungs. The left ventricle is the lower chamber of the left side of the heart, which pumps arterial oxygenated blood out through the aorta to the tissues of the body*

■ **cardiac pacemaker:** *an electric apparatus used for maintaining a normal sinus rhythm of myocardial contraction by electrically stimulating the heart muscle;* also known as a pacemaker

■ **blood pressure:** *the pressure exerted by the circulating volume of blood on the wall of the arteries, the veins, and the chambers of the heart. The pressure in the aorta and the large arteries of a healthy young adult is approximately 120 mm Hg during systole and 80 mm Hg in diastole*

electrical signal is spread through the right and left **atria.** These muscular chambers then contract and empty their blood into the right and left **ventricles.** The electrical signal is briefly held in the AV node while the atria are contracting. The signal then travels from the AV node to the bundle of His, both bundle branches, and the Purkinje fibers. Both ventricles then contract and pump their blood out to the lungs and body. This pumping action must happen throughout life to deliver oxygen-rich blood to the body and remove carbon dioxide gas from the tissues. Like the lungs, the proper functioning of the heart is vital for life. Because of this importance, the heart has more than one signal-generating area. If the sinoatrial node is damaged and not signaling properly, the atrioventricular node will send out signals. The rate is slower than from the SA node, but fast enough for most activities. If the AV node should also fail, the bundle of His and Purkinje fibers will send out their own signals. However, this rate is too slow for good health. People with this condition are often fitted with a **cardiac pacemaker** that signals a faster heart rate that allows normal activity.

The heart has two separate pumping halves (Figure 1-20). The right side of the heart pumps blood to the lungs (*pulmonary circulation*). The left side of the heart pumps blood to the body (*systemic circulation*). Each half is discussed in turn. By the end of the presentation you should be able to trace the flow of blood through the body, lungs, and heart. When the heart pumps blood through the pulmonary and circulatory systems, there is an increase in the **blood pressure.** The higher pressure found when the heart contracts is called the *systolic pressure.* After the heart contracts, it rests for a short time period. The blood pressure then drops to a resting level, which is called the *diastolic pressure.* When measuring blood pressure it is important to find both the systolic and diastolic pressures. These are recorded as the systolic over the diastolic; for example, 120/80 millimeters of mercury (mm Hg) pressure. Table 1-2 lists the normal ranges for blood pressure for three age ranges of patients.

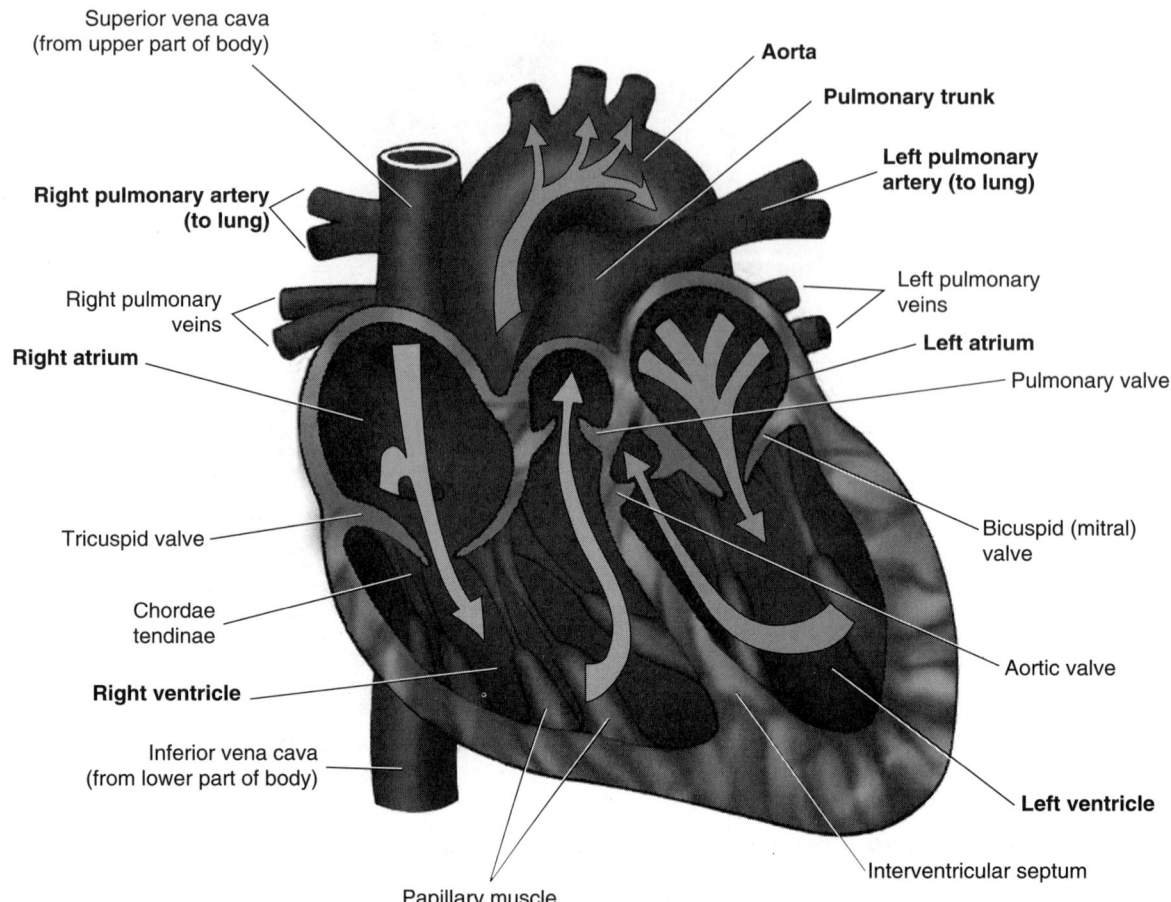

Superior vena cava
(from upper part of body)

Aorta

Pulmonary trunk

**Left pulmonary
artery (to lung)**

**Right pulmonary artery
(to lung)**

Left pulmonary
veins

Right pulmonary
veins

Left atrium

Right atrium

Pulmonary valve

Tricuspid valve

Bicuspid (mitral)
valve

Chordae
tendinae

Aortic valve

Right ventricle

Inferior vena cava
(from lower part of body)

Left ventricle

Interventricular septum

Papillary muscle

Figure 1-20   Interior, front view of the heart showing the structures and blood flow. The unoxygenated blood returning from the body and going to the lungs is shown by the white arrows. The oxygenated blood returning from the lungs and going to the body is shown by the dark arrows.

■ ***venule:*** *any one of the small blood vessels that gather blood from the capillary bed and come together to form the veins*

■ ***vein:*** *one of the many vessels that convey blood from the capillaries to the heart. The systemic veins carry blood to the right atrium of the heart; the pulmonary veins carry blood to the left atrium of the heart*

■ ***artery*** *(plural,* ***arteries***): *one of the large blood vessels carrying blood in a direction away from the heart*

Pulmonary Circulation

The right side of the heart and related structures are discussed first. Let us start by tracing the path of blood from capillaries in the head and feet. (Refer to Figures 1-20 and 1-21 as you follow what happens to the blood.) The capillaries are the smallest blood vessels, with very thin walls. It is easy for oxygen from the blood to diffuse into the tissues and for waste carbon dioxide gas to diffuse out of the tissues and into the blood. The blood from the head and feet is pushed along by other blood circulating behind it. It enters small **venules** and then larger **veins.** The blood from the feet enters the large vein called the inferior vena cava within the abdomen. The blood from the head (and arms) enters into the superior vena cava. All of the blood is then emptied into the right atrium. When the atrium contracts, the blood is forced through the tricuspid valve and into the right ventricle. The tricuspid valve separates the two right heart chambers. It is designed like a one-way valve and only allows blood to flow from the right atrium to the right ventricle. Chordae tendineae and papillary muscles prevent the valve from collapsing backward and letting blood leak from the lower to the upper chamber. When the right ventricle contracts, the blood is pumped through the pulmonary valve and into the pulmonary **artery.** The pulmonary valve is also designed only to let the blood flow out of the right ventricle. The main pulmonary artery splits to carry blood to both lungs. The right pulmonary artery branch carries blood to the right lung and the left pulmonary artery branch carries blood to the left lung. As with the repeated branchings of the tracheobronchial tree, the pulmonary arteries subdivide repeatedly. The right

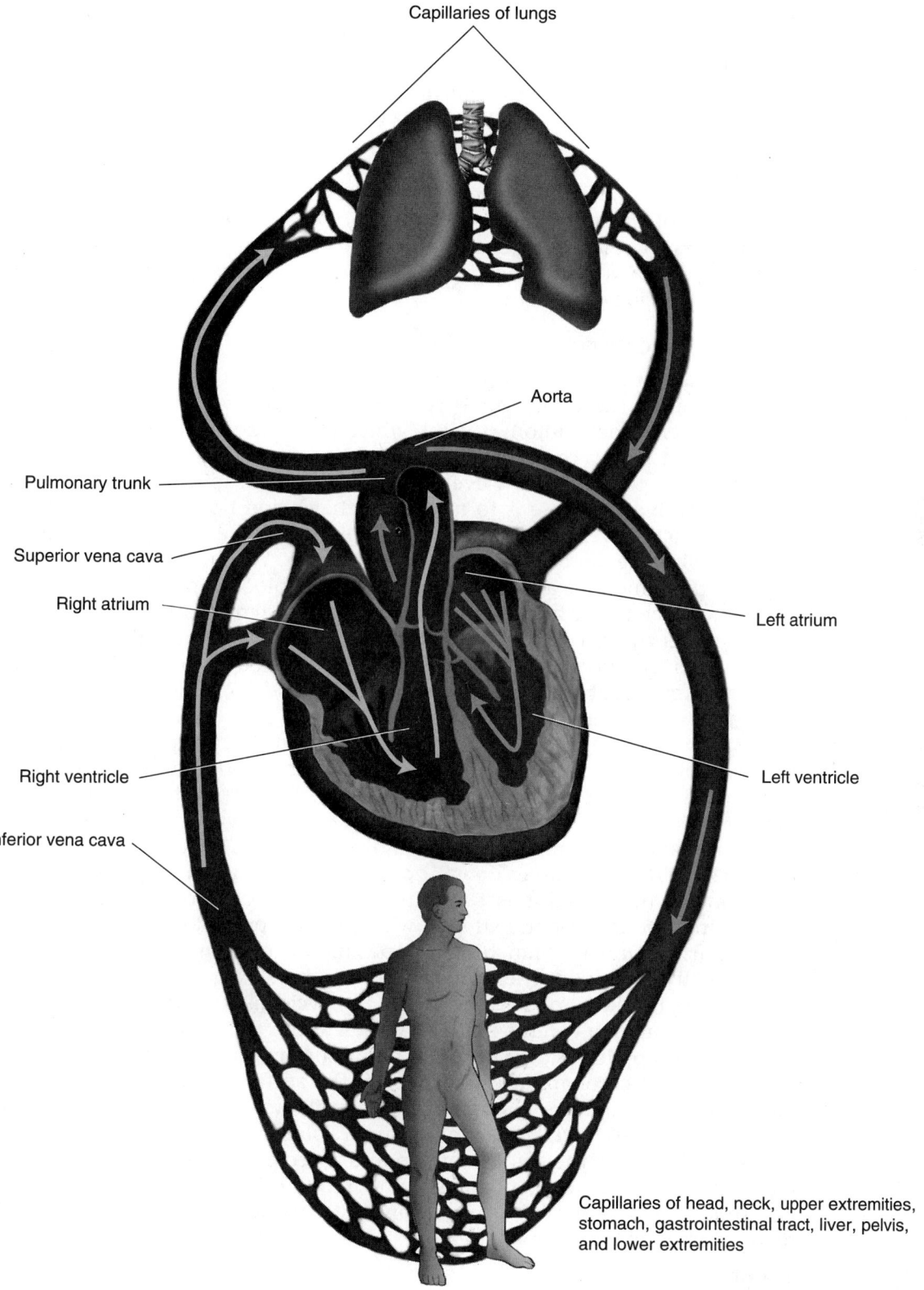

Capillaries of lungs

Aorta

Pulmonary trunk

Superior vena cava

Right atrium

Left atrium

Right ventricle

Left ventricle

Inferior vena cava

Capillaries of head, neck, upper extremities, stomach, gastrointestinal tract, liver, pelvis, and lower extremities

Figure 1-21   Schematic drawing of the pulmonary and systemic circulations. Unoxygenated blood from the body returns to the right side of the heart before going to the lungs. Oxygenated blood returns from the lungs to the left side of the heart before going to the body.

■ *arteriole:* the smallest vascular branch of the arterial circulation

pulmonary artery splits into three lobar arteries—one for each of the three lobes. These three lobar arteries then split into ten segmental arteries. The left pulmonary artery splits into two lobar arteries—one for each lobe. These two lobar arteries then divide into eight segmental arteries. (Review Figure 1-8.) These segmental arteries continue to divide to **arterioles.** The final vessels are the pulmonary capillaries. They are thin walled and allow easy diffusion of oxygen from the alveoli into the blood and carbon dioxide from the blood into the alveoli (see Figure 1-9). The pulmonary capillaries cover about 85% to 95% of the surface area of the alveoli. The oxygenated blood in the pulmonary capillaries then gathers in small and then larger veins. Eventually it collects in the two right lung and two left lung pulmonary veins. This oxygenated blood then enters the left side of the heart.

Systemic Circulation

The left side of the heart pumps blood out to the body. Let us follow this blood flow starting in the lungs. After exchanging oxygen for carbon dioxide, the blood collects in the pulmonary veins, which return the blood to the left atrium. When the left atrium contracts (at the same time as the right atrium), the blood flows through the bicuspid valve (also known as the mitral valve; see Figure 1-20). The valve's purpose is to make sure that blood flows only from the left atrium to the left ventricle. Like the tricuspid valve, the bicuspid valve is supported by chordae tendineae and papillary muscles. When the left ventricle contracts (at the same time as the right ventricle), the blood is pumped out through the aortic valve to the aorta. The aortic valve is designed only to let blood out of the left ventricle. The blood in the aorta is distributed through progressively smaller arteries and arterioles to the tissues of the body. Several large arteries come off the aorta at the arch (Figure 1-17, 1-18, and 1-21). The right subclavian artery goes to the right shoulder area and turns into the right brachial artery as it goes to the right arm. The right common carotid artery supplies blood to the right side of the head and brain. The left common carotid artery supplies blood to the left side of the head and brain. The left subclavian artery sends blood to the left shoulder and turns into the left brachial artery to supply the left arm. Both brachial arteries split into radial and ulnar arteries to supply blood to each hand. The aorta then curves down into the body. Numerous arteries branch off to supply the intercostal muscles, kidneys, intestine, and so on. The aorta ends by splitting into the femoral arteries, which then supply blood to the legs. Each femoral artery and its branchings supply blood to the respective leg (Figure 1-18). Finally, the blood enters the capillaries, where oxygen is given off and carbon dioxide is taken on. This completes the cycle, as the unoxygenated blood returns to venules and veins on its way back to the right side of the heart.

The heart supplies its own needs for blood through two coronary arteries (Figure 1-17). Both coronary arteries come off the aorta just past the aortic valve. Blood flows through the arteries during diastole when the heart is at rest. The left coronary artery and its branchings supply blood to most of the left ventricle and some blood to the right ventricle and interventricular septum. The right coronary artery and its branchings supply blood to most of the right ventricle and some blood to the left ventricle and interventricular septum. The heart's deoxygenated blood enters its venous system through the right atrium.

Shunt

■ *shunt:* a diversion of blood from one side of the heart to the other that bypasses the pulmonary circulation; also called left-to-right shunt or right-to-left shunt

As discussed earlier, blood that passes through the right heart goes through the lungs to be reoxygenated. However, normally a small amount bypasses the lung tissues. This is referred to as an anatomic **shunt** (Figure 1-22). Shunted blood leaves the right side of the heart, misses contact with any alveoli, and is returned to the left side of the heart unoxygenated (Figure 1-22B). This shunted blood is mainly from the bronchi, cardiac veins, and pleura. Any blood that has bypassed the alveoli remains low in oxygen. The shunted blood rejoins reoxygenated blood to go out to the body. Usually this small drop in the oxygen level is not a

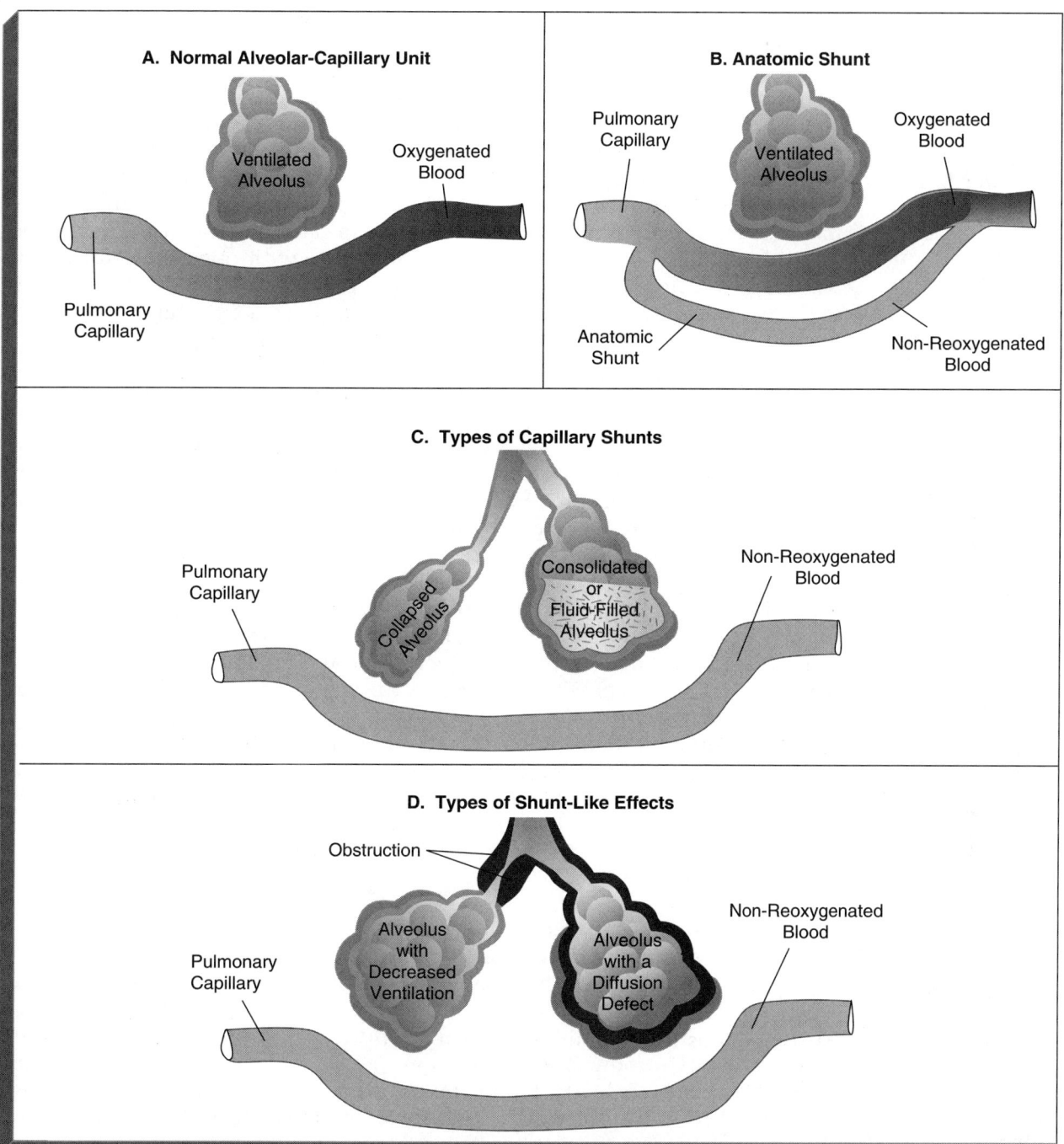

Figure 1-22 Pulmonary shunting. A. Normal alveolar-capillary unit. B. Anatomic shunt. C. Types of capillary shunts. D. Types of shunt-like effects.

problem. However, a number of lung diseases can dangerously increase the amount of shunted blood. These are shown in Figures 1-22C and D and are discussed in Chapter 2. Additionally, a hole between the heart chambers will let blood flow incorrectly and cause a shunt.

Vital Signs: Heart Rate, Blood Pressure, and Respiratory Rate

The vital signs of heart rate, blood pressure, and respiratory rate are used to evaluate a person's basic cardiopulmonary condition. When the vital signs are found to be in the expected range, we have indications that the patient's breathing and circulatory systems are working as expected. When one or more of the vital signs

■■■ **Note:** *If a pulse cannot be found, call for help immediately. Evaluate the patient's breathing. If he or she is not breathing and/or has no pulse, begin cardiopulmonary resuscitation efforts.* ■■

■ **blood:** *the liquid pumped by the heart through all the arteries, veins, and capillaries. The blood is composed of a clear yellow fluid, called plasma; the formed elements, erythrocytes and leukocytes; and a series of cell types with different functions*

■ **plasma:** *the watery, straw-colored, fluid portion of the lymph and blood in which the leukocytes, erythrocytes, and platelets are suspended*

■ **erythrocyte:** *a biconcave, disk-shaped cell that contains hemoglobin. The major cellular element of the circulating blood, its principal function is to transport oxygen and carbon dioxide*

■ **leukocyte:** *a white blood cell, one of the formed elements of the circulating blood system. Five types of leukocytes are classified by the presence or absence of granules in the cytoplasm of the cell. Leukocytes are able to squeeze through intracellular spaces to engulf and destroy invading bacteria, fungi, viruses, and toxic proteins from allergic reactions or cellular injury*

■ **thrombocyte:** *a disk- or plate-like structure that is the smallest of the formed blood elements. It does not have a nucleus. Because of its very fragile membrane, it tends to stick to damaged or uneven surfaces. This causes the other blood elements to adhere to it, forming a blood clot. Also called a* platelet

are not as expected, we have indications of a problem. The nurse or RCP should be called to further evaluate the patient.

When counting any patient's heart rate, it important to count it for a reasonable time period of 30 to 60 seconds. This is because the heart rate may vary; counting for less time will not give an accurate value. The standard is to record the heart rate in beats per minute. Obviously, if the rate is counted for 30 seconds, it must be doubled for a minute count. It is acceptable to count the heart rate at any of the sites shown in Figure 1-18. Depending on your institution, you may also be trained to check the pulse at the apical site of the heart. Remember that this is the point of strongest heartbeat that is felt through the chest wall to the left of the sternum. Most commonly the pulse is counted at the radial site in the wrist. If the pulse is weak at this site, check the patient's carotid site in the neck. A carotid artery can be located on either side of the larynx.

The respiratory rate should also be reported in breaths per minute. Again, this can be done either by counting for 60 seconds or by counting for 30 seconds and doubling the value. The respiratory rate is usually counted by looking at the patient's chest and/or abdomen rise and fall as he or she breathes. If the patient's breathing is shallow, you may need to place your hand on his or her upper chest area or abdomen to feel each breath. One breath includes an inspiration and an expiration. It is usually easiest to check the respiratory rate by starting on an inspiration and on exhalation counting the breath. Table 1-2 shows the normal resting respiratory rate for three age ranges of patients. Notify the nurse, RCP, or supervisor if your patient is found to have a respiratory rate that is unexpectedly higher or lower than that listed or has an unusual breathing pattern.

The blood pressure is recorded as the systolic and diastolic pressures measured from either arm. It is possible to measure the blood pressure from a leg if necessary. If you are unsure about the sound you hear or the reading you see on the blood pressure unit, take the blood pressure again. Table 1-2 shows the normal resting blood pressure for three age ranges of patients. Notify the nurse, RCP, or supervisor if your patient is found to have a blood pressure that is unexpectedly higher or lower than that listed.

■■■ BLOOD

Blood is the liquid substance that is vitally important for ensuring that the cells of the body are supplied with the substances needed to keep them alive. Blood is normally found only within the blood vessels. As noted earlier, blood carries oxygen from the lungs to the body tissues and carbon dioxide from the tissues to the lungs. Additionally, blood carries nutrients throughout the body and removes waste products for excretion. Most medications are distributed throughout the body by the blood and circulatory system. Blood is composed of the following four components: **plasma, erythrocytes, leukocytes,** and **thrombocytes.**

Plasma

Plasma is the watery part of blood. It is what remains after all of the blood cells have been removed. Plasma is about 90% water. The other 10% is made up of proteins, electrolytes, nutrients, hormones, vitamins, and waste products. They give plasma its light yellow color. Besides adding volume to maintain the blood pressure, plasma acts as a vehicle to carry the blood cells and other substances throughout the body. Oxygen and carbon dioxide easily diffuse back and forth among the lungs, plasma, erythrocytes, and body cells. Only a small amount of these gases actually stays in the plasma.

Erythrocytes

Erythrocytes are also called red blood cells (RBCs) because of their reddish coloration. Normally, between 42% and 45% of the total volume of blood is made

■ *hematocrit:* a measure of the packed cell volume of red cells, expressed as a percentage of the total blood volume

■ *hemoglobin:* a complex protein-iron compound in the erythrocyte that carries oxygen to the cells from the lungs and carbon dioxide away from the cells to the lungs

■ *iron (Fe):* a common metallic element essential for the synthesis of hemoglobin

■ *carbon monoxide:* a colorless, odorless, poisonous gas produced by the combustion of carbon or organic fuels in a limited oxygen supply, as in the cylinders of an internal combustion engine. Carbon monoxide combines very strongly with hemoglobin, preventing the formation of oxyhemoglobin and reducing the oxygen supply to the tissues. Prolonged exposure to high levels of carbon monoxide can result in death

■ *allergen:* a substance that can produce a hypersensitive reaction in the body but is not necessarily harmful by itself. Some common allergens are bacteria, pollen, animal dander, house dust, feathers, and various foods

■ *allergic:* having an allergy; having a hypersensitive reaction to basically harmless antigens, most of which are found in the environment

■ *antibodies:* immunoglobins produced by lymphocytes in response to an antigen such as bacteria, viruses, or other common substances. An antibody is specific to an antigen

■ *antigen:* a substance, usually a bacterium or foreign protein, that causes the formation of an antibody and reacts specifically with that antibody

up of erythrocytes. This laboratory value is called the patient's **hematocrit.** New erythrocytes are constantly being made in several bones of the body. Old RBCs are removed by the spleen and liver. Erythrocytes are vitally important because they carry the large majority of the oxygen and carbon dioxide between the lungs and body's cells (Figure 1-23). These gases are able to temporarily bind to **hemoglobin** molecules found within the erythrocytes. Hemoglobin is a large protein that makes up most of the RBC. **Iron (Fe)** is one of the key components of hemoglobin. Specifically, it is the iron within the hemoglobin that picks up the oxygen and carbon dioxide. When oxygen combines with hemoglobin, the RBC takes on its characteristic bright red color. After the RBC has given up its oxygen to the tissues, the color changes to a darker red. Besides these two gases, hemoglobin will also bind with the poisonous gas **carbon monoxide.** When this happens, the hemoglobin cannot carry any oxygen. Because of this, death can be caused by exposure to too much carbon monoxide.

Leukocytes

Leukocytes are also called white blood cells (WBCs) because of their white color. WBCs are one of the most important defenses against invading bacteria. They also protect the body from other harmful substances. There are five different types of leukocytes:

1. Neutrophils—mainly responsible for killing invading bacteria
2. Eosinophils—primary cells responsible for fighting the **allergen** that causes an **allergic** reaction
3. Basophils—secondary cells for fighting allergens
4. Monocytes—secondary cells for fighting invading bacteria during a chronic infection
5. Lymphocytes—produce **antibodies** that inactivate **antigens** to prevent a second infection by the same bacteria or other organism

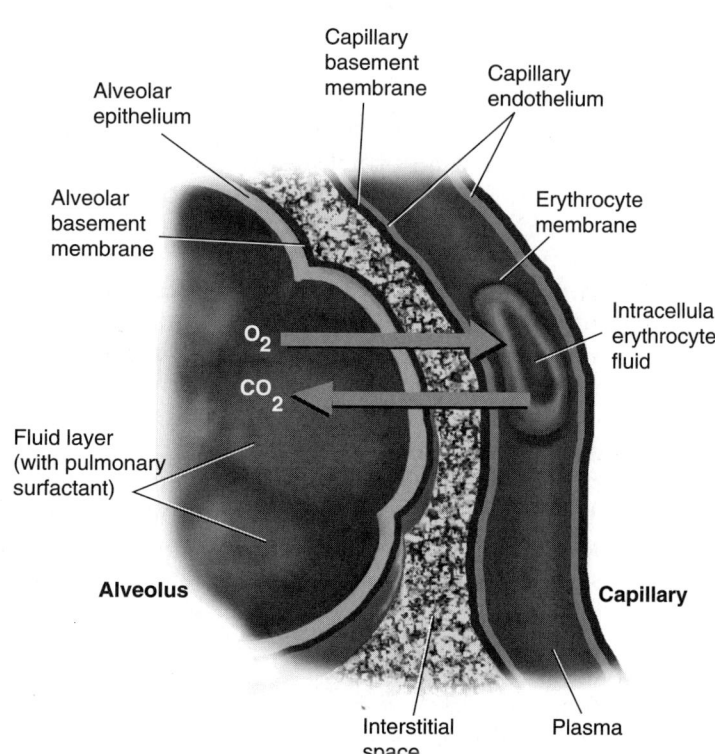

ALVEOLAR-CAPILLARY MEMBRANE

Figure 1-23 The alveolar-capillary membrane through which oxygen and carbon dioxide diffuse. Only the alveolus, interstitial space, and capillary endothelium separate the gases from the blood.

When trying to determine the health of a person's immune system, the physician often orders a blood sample taken to count how many of each type of leukocyte are found (called a *differential count*). Often this information is very helpful in understanding the type of infection and how the body is responding to it. Also, some patients, such as those with AIDS, have immune systems that are not functioning properly.

Thrombocytes

Thrombocytes are often called platelets because they are shaped like small disks or plates. They are the smallest of the three blood components. Unlike erythrocytes and leukocytes, platelets are not true cells, because they lack a nucleus. The platelets are formed in red bone marrow. They are designed to cause blood to **clot** after a cut or other injury. Platelets have a thin membrane that sticks to any rough surface area. Erythrocytes then stick to the platelets and form a clot. Without them, even the smallest cut would not stop bleeding. Often a laboratory test (called a *clotting time*) is performed to check the time it takes a blood sample to clot. There are disease conditions that cause blood either to clot too quickly or to take too long to clot. Either situation can be very dangerous. Blood that clots too quickly can actually clot within the blood vessels. This most often happens in the lower leg veins. If blood takes too long to clot, cuts will bleed longer than expected. Obviously, this would be a problem in a patient who is having surgery or giving a blood sample.

■ **clot:** *a semisolid, gelatinous mass; the end result of the clotting process of blood. Red cells, white cells, and platelets are enmeshed in an insoluble fibrin network of the blood clot*

■■■■ VENTILATION AND RESPIRATION

All of the preceding discussion in this chapter has dealt with the cardiopulmonary and related organ systems. They enable the body to do two crucial things: first, get oxygen from the air to the tissues and body cells, and second, remove carbon dioxide from the body. In order for these two things to take place, all of the previously discussed systems must work properly. Altogether they result in ventilation and respiration—two separate things that normally work together. Ventilation and respiration are presented separately here for easier understanding.

Ventilation

■ **ventilation:** *the process by which gases are moved into and out of the lungs*

Ventilation is the act of moving air into and out of the lungs. Simply put, this is breathing. For a normal, resting inspiration to take place, the following steps must occur. The respiratory center of the brain must sense the presence of carbon dioxide. A nerve signal must travel from the respiratory center down the phrenic nerve to the diaphragm. Other nerve signals from the brain go to the throat muscles, to keep the airway open, and to accessory inspiratory muscles. The muscles must be functioning normally and contract when they receive the nerve signals. Stimulation of the inspiratory muscles causes them to contract and enlarge the thorax. This expands the size of the lungs. This lung expansion causes a drop in the gas pressure within the lungs. Outside air is then drawn into the lungs to fill the increased space.

After the lungs have filled, stretch-sensitive nerves in the chest wall and lungs are stimulated. These signal to the respiratory center to stop inspiration. When this happens, the inspiratory muscles relax. The lungs, ribs, and abdominal contents then go back to their previous resting position. This causes the lungs to become smaller. Provided that the airway remains open, the smaller lungs push out some of the air that they had previously inspired. This is expiration/ exhalation.

When observing someone's breathing, it is important to note the rate, the depth, and the pattern. These three things should be looked at individually and together. A number of factors influence each one and all three interact with each other. As discussed earlier, the respiratory center of the medulla oblongata normally determines the respiratory rate. The carbon dioxide level is a key influence. In some cases, a low oxygen level in the blood (hypoxemia) will be the main stimulus to breathe.

Figure 1-24 illustrates several issues affecting depth and pattern of breathing. The average adult male inhales a resting volume of about 500 mL. This resting volume is called the **tidal volume (V_T or VT).** Of this 500 mL tidal volume, only the first 350 mL reach the alveoli for gas exchange. The first 150 mL to reach the alveoli come from the upper airway dead space. Additionally, about 200 mL of fresh outside air are inhaled and reach the alveoli. The last 150 mL of inhaled outside air remain in the airways. With exhalation, the 150 mL of gas in the airways are exhaled along with 200 mL of gas from the alveoli. The last 150 mL of exhaled gas remain in the airways as dead space gas. This pattern of rebreathing some "old" air from the airways with some fresh air repeats itself with every breath. (If you think it is strange to rebreathe 150 mL of air, think of the poor giraffe with its long neck!)

These tidal volume values are for an average adult male. Obviously, the actual tidal volume and dead space volume for each person, adult and child, will depend on how large the person is, but the principles are still the same. The pattern of breathing at rest, with a normal tidal volume and a normal rate, is also shown in Figure 1-24. As can be seen, inspiration takes about half as much time as exhalation and the pause before the next breath in. This normal rate, tidal volume, and breathing pattern is called **eupnea.**

■ *tidal volume (V_T or TV):* the amount of air inhaled and exhaled during normal ventilation

■ *eupnea: normal breathing*

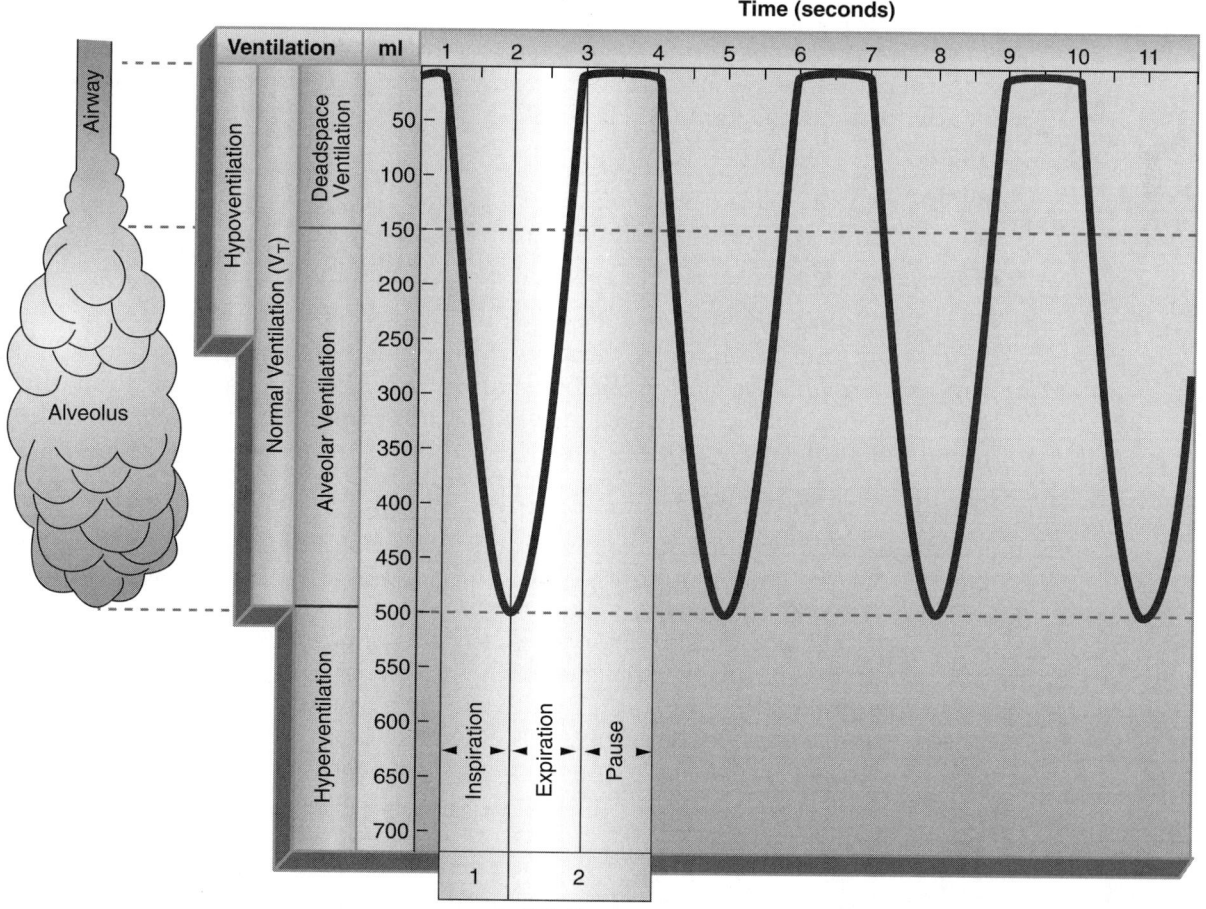

Figure 1-24 Normal, spontaneous breathing depth and pattern for an adult (eupnea). Hypoventilation (shallow breathing) and hyperventilation (deep breathing) are also shown.

■ *respiration:* the process of the molecular exchange of oxygen and carbon dioxide within the body's tissues, from the lungs to cellular oxidation processes

Obviously, not all patients breathe normally. Inhaling a smaller than normal volume can lead to hypoventilation. This is shown by a high carbon dioxide level, produced because the alveoli are not being ventilated deeply enough. Breathing a larger than normal tidal volume can lead to hyperventilation. This is shown by a low carbon dioxide level, produced because the alveoli are being overventilated.

Respiration

Respiration is the act of moving oxygen and carbon dioxide between the blood and the cells of the body. It is made up of two separate stages: external respiration and internal respiration. *External respiration* involves the exchange of oxygen and carbon dioxide between the atmosphere and the blood. For it to take place, the following are needed:

■ Effective alveolar ventilation (as described earlier)
■ Normal alveolar-capillary membrane (Figure 1-23)
■ Blood with normal erythrocytes and plasma present in the pulmonary capillaries
■ Normal pumping of blood by the heart through the lungs and body

If all of these things are present, carbon dioxide will diffuse from the blood into the lungs to be exhaled. This will allow the blood to pick up oxygen from the fresh, inhaled air. The heart will then pump the oxygenated blood throughout the body.

Internal respiration involves the use of oxygen by the body's cells and production of the waste gas carbon dioxide. Internal respiration is the ultimate purpose of ventilation and external respiration. It is in the cells of the body that oxygen is used for metabolic purposes to keep a person alive, generate new cells, and carry on all life-related chemical reactions. For internal respiration to take place, the following are needed:

■ Effective alveolar ventilation
■ Effective external respiration
■ Diffusion of oxygen from the erythrocytes into the cells
■ Functioning cells to use the oxygen for metabolic processes
■ Diffusion of waste carbon dioxide out of the cells into the blood

If the brain, nerves, muscles, airways, lungs, heart, blood, and blood vessels work as intended, the cells of the body will receive the oxygen and carbon dioxide will be eliminated. The elegance with which the body is able to do all of these interconnected, intricate steps is a wondrous thing.

Blood Gas Values and Acid-Base Balance

Because of their importance, oxygen and carbon dioxide levels are frequently measured in patients. One test requires the drawing of a sample of blood from an artery. This blood sample is taken to the laboratory for measurement of oxygen, carbon dioxide, acid-base level, and some other related values. The test is called an *arterial blood gas sample* or *ABG*.

Another procedure for measuring the patient's oxygen level involves a device called a *pulse oximeter.* Put simply, it is able to measure how full of oxygen the erythrocytes are. The pulse oximeter does this by measuring special light levels that shine through the skin and blood. When a pulse oximeter is used on a patient, arterial blood gas samples may not have to be taken as often. The pulse oximeter may be used temporarily and then removed or left on the patient for an extended period to continuously monitor the patient. If it is left on the patient, a low oxygen level alarm is usually set. The role of the patient care technician in caring for patients having either test performed is discussed in Chapter 3.

REVIEW QUESTIONS

Multiple Choice Questions

1. The pulmonary lymphatic system
   a. Adds fluid to the alveoli.
   b. Adds fluid to the pleural space.
   c. Removes erythrocytes from around the alveoli.
   d. Removes fluid from around the alveoli.

2. All of the following are chambers of the heart EXCEPT the
   a. Central ventricle.
   b. Right ventricle.
   c. Left ventricle.
   d. Right atrium.
   e. Left atrium.

3. All of the following structures are needed to form speech:
   1. Tongue   a. 1, 3
   2. Nasal passage   b. 3, 5
   3. Vocal cords   c. 1, 2, 3
   4. Esophagus   d. 1, 2, 3, 4, 5
   5. Trachea

4. Shunt would best be defined as
   a. Ventilation without blood flow through the lungs.
   b. Neither blood flow nor ventilation through the lungs.
   c. Blood flow through the lungs without the opportunity for gas exchange.
   d. Matching of blood flow through the lungs with ventilation.

5. The right lung has ____ lobes and the left lung has ____ lobes.
   a. 2, 3
   b. 10, 8
   c. 8, 10
   d. 3, 2

6. The purpose of the fluid between the pleural membranes is
   a. To allow the lungs and chest wall to easily move over each other during breathing.
   b. To protect the lungs from inhaled bacteria.
   c. To allow oxygen and carbon dioxide to easily diffuse.
   d. To hold the lungs in their proper shape.

7. Internal respiration involves
   1. Oxygen diffusing from the blood into   a. 1, 4
      the cells of the body   b. 3, 5
   2. Carbon dioxide diffusing into the cells c. 4, 5
      of the body   d. 2, 3
   3. Oxygen diffusing into the blood from
      the lungs
   4. Carbon dioxide diffusing into the
      blood from the cells of the body
   5. Carbon dioxide diffusing from the
      blood into the lungs

8. Normal blood pressure of an adult would be
   a. 100/70 mm Hg.
   b. 120/80 cm water.
   c. 60/20 mm Hg.
   d. 120/80 mm Hg.
   e. 100/70 cm water.

9. All of the following are purposes of the pulmonary system except
   a. Bringing oxygen to the cells of the body.
   b. Removing carbon dioxide from the body.
   c. Bringing oxygen into the body.

10. What is the purpose of surfactant?
    a. Surfactant reduces the amount of work the heart has to perform to pump blood.
    b. Surfactant reduces the surface tension of water in the lungs.
    c. Surfactant kills bacteria and other pathogens that enter the alveoli.
    d. Surfactant increases the surface tension of water in the lungs.
    e. Inhaled dust and bacteria get caught in the surfactant that lines the airways.

11. What role does oxygen play in stimulating breathing?
    a. Breathing is stimulated when a low oxygen level is sensed by the central chemoreceptors.
    b. Breathing is decreased when a low oxygen level is sensed by the central chemoreceptors.
    c. Breathing is stimulated when a low oxygen level is sensed by the peripheral chemoreceptors.
    d. Breathing is not affected by a person's oxygen level.

12. Tidal volume is
    a. The volume of oxygen taken into the body during a normal breath.
    b. The maximum volume that can be inhaled.
    c. The volume of gas that would be breathed during heavy exercise.
    d. The volume of gas a resting person normally breathes.
    e. The volume of carbon dioxide that the body exhales with each breath.

13. Which of the following is the correct flow of blood through the heart and lungs, starting with the lungs?
    a. Right atrium, right ventricle, lungs, left atrium, left ventricle, body
    b. Right atrium, left atrium, right ventricle, left ventricle, body
    c. Left atrium, left ventricle, body, right atrium, right ventricle, lungs
    d. Left atrium, left ventricle, lungs, right atrium, right ventricle, body

14. The alveolar-capillary membrane is composed of
    a. Alveolar type II cells, interstitium, capillary bed.

b. Macrophages, alveolar type II cells, interstitium, capillary bed.

c. Alveolar type I cells, interstitium, capillary bed.

d. Alveolar type I and type II cells, pulmonary arteries, macrophages.

15. The normal breathing pattern (eupnea) is
   a. Pause, inspiration, and expiration so that the timing is inspiration of about 1 second and expiration of about 2 seconds.
   b. Inspiration, expiration, and pause so that the timing is pause and inspiration of about 1 second and expiration and pause of about 2 seconds.
   c. Pause, inspiration, and expiration so that the timing is pause and inspiration of about 2 seconds and expiration of about 1 second.
   d. Inspiration, pause, and expiration so that the timing is inspiration of about 2 seconds and pause and expiration of about 1 second.

16. All of the following are conducting airways except
   a. Alveolar ducts.
   b. Terminal bronchioles.
   c. Segmental bronchi.
   d. Bronchioles.

17. The hemidiaphragms are stimulated by
   a. Cervical nerves.
   b. Intercostal nerves.
   c. Vagus nerve.
   d. Phrenic nerves.
   e. Glossopharyngeal nerve.

18. Dead space can be defined as
   a. Blood flow through the lungs without matching ventilation.
   b. Matching of blood flow and ventilation through the lungs.
   c. Inhaled volume that does not reach the alveoli.
   d. The volume of air found in the sinuses, nose, and mouth.

19. Which of the following carries most of the oxygen throughout the body?
   a. Erythrocytes
   b. Plasma
   c. Platelets/thrombocytes
   d. Leukocytes

20. All of the following are valves of the heart except
   a. Aortic valve.
   b. Pyloric valve.
   c. Tricuspid valve.
   d. Pulmonary valve.
   e. Bicuspid valve.

21. The nose conditions inspired air in all of the following ways EXCEPT
   a. Warms cold air to body temperature.
   b. Dries the air.
   c. Cools hot air to body temperature.
   d. Filters the air.
   e. Humidifies the air.

22. Which of the following are found within the mediastinum?
   1. Heart   **a.** 1, 2, 3
   2. Stomach   **b.** 1, 3, 4

3. Esophagus   **c.** 3, 4
4. Trachea   **d.** 1, 2, 3, 4, 5
5. Larynx

23. As blood flows through the right side of the heart, it is _____ in oxygen and as it flows through the left side of the heart it is _____ in oxygen.
   a. Low, high
   b. High, low
   c. High, high
   d. Low, low

24. The normal resting breathing rate for an older child is
   a. 12–20/minute.
   b. 22–30/minute.
   c. 20–24/minute.
   d. 30–60/minute.

25. What role does carbon dioxide have in stimulating breathing?
   a. A low carbon dioxide level in the brain stimulates breathing.
   b. A high carbon dioxide level in the brain stimulates breathing.
   c. A high carbon dioxide level in the brain decreases breathing.
   d. A low carbon dioxide level in the peripheral chemoreceptors stimulates breathing.
   e. Carbon dioxide level has no effect on breathing, only oxygen level.

26. The lower airway is protected from inhalation (aspiration) of foreign matter by the
   a. Tongue.
   b. Vocal cords.
   c. Mucociliary escalator.
   d. Epiglottis.
   e. Carina.

27. Gases are exchanged mainly through which of the following structures?
   a. Alveolar-capillary membrane
   b. Terminal bronchioles
   c. Respiratory bronchioles
   d. Glottis

28. The heart supplies blood to itself through the
   1. Aorta   **a.** 1
   2. Pulmonary arteries   **b.** 3, 5
   3. Right coronary artery   **c.** 1, 2
   4. Central coronary artery   **d.** 3, 4, 5
   5. Left coronary artery   **e.** 1, 2, 3, 4, 5

29. All of the following are roles of the rib cage in breathing EXCEPT
   a. Recoil to aid expiration.
   b. Expand out to aid inspiration.
   c. Offer support to the trachea and mainstem bronchi.
   d. Protect the lungs and heart.

30. The normal pacemaker of the heart is/are the
   a. Purkinje fibers.
   b. Sinoatrial (SA) node.
   c. Bundle of His.
   d. Atrioventricular (AV) node.

31. What is the purpose of the mucociliary escalator?
   a. To prevent the inhalation (aspiration) of foreign matter
   b. To trap and remove inhaled dust and particles
   c. To move phagocytes from the alveoli to the pharynx
   d. To move phagocytes from the pharynx to the alveoli

32. The primary muscles of breathing are the
   a. Hemidiaphragms.
   b. Internal intercostal muscles.
   c. External intercostal muscles.
   d. Sternocleidomastoid muscles.
   e. Abdominal muscles.

33. The alveoli are protected from infection by the
   a. Mucociliary cells.
   b. Type I cells.
   c. Kohn cells.
   d. Macrophages.
   e. Goblet cells.

CHAPTER 2

Selected Cardiopulmonary Diseases

OBJECTIVES:

After reading this chapter, you will be able to:

- *Identify certain cardiopulmonary diseases.*
- *Identify the clinical presentation of certain cardiopulmonary diseases.*
- *Identify the etiology of certain cardiopulmonary diseases.*
- *Identify the procedures used to diagnose certain cardiopulmonary diseases.*
- *Identify how certain cardiopulmonary diseases are treated.*
- *Identify the prognosis for patients who have certain cardiopulmonary diseases.*

OVERVIEW

This chapter briefly covers selected, common diseases that affect the lungs, heart, and related systems. You can refer to Chapter 1 as needed to review normal anatomy. Before starting, it is important that you understand what disease is.

Disease can be defined as a specific illness or disorder having a characteristic set of signs and symptoms. The illness or disorder causes the abnormal function of a structure (example: broken nose), part (example: defective heart valve), system (example: asthma), or the whole of the organism (example: bloodborne infection). The disease may be caused by heredity, infection, diet, or environment, or a combination of these factors. **Signs** are objective evidence, found by an examiner, of disease or dysfunction. Often one or more specific signs are associated with a specific disease. For example, a productive cough usually accompanies bronchitis or pneumonia. **Symptoms** are subjective indications of a disease or change in condition as felt by the patient. For example, patients with heart and/or lung disease often say they are short of breath.

This chapter briefly discusses some of the key aspects of selected, common cardiopulmonary and related system diseases. Consult the patient's physician, nurse, respiratory care practitioner, or more detailed written material for additional information as needed. It is important to remember that all of the diseases covered here can interfere with the patient's breathing and/or heart function. Because of this, most patients with these problems will have a lower than normal oxygen level. Some of these diseases can lead to a patient's rapid deterioration and even death. Always be vigilant in monitoring your patient's breathing and heart function! Report any change in condition to the physician, nurse, or respiratory care practitioner. Remember that stopping of breathing or heart function for only 4 to 6 minutes can result in irreversible brain damage or death.

To begin to understand these diseases, you must understand these key words: **etiology, diagnose, diagnosis, treatment,** and **prognosis.**

PULMONARY SYSTEM PROBLEMS: UPPER (LARGER) AIRWAY

Upper airway problems, such as infection, are experienced by almost everyone at some point in their lives. They are unpleasant but rarely truly dangerous.

■ **disease:** *a specific illness or disorder having a characteristic set of signs and symptoms*

■ **signs:** *objective evidence of disease or dysfunction; vital signs include measurements of blood pressure, pulse, and respiration rate*

■ **symptoms:** *changes felt by the patient (in his or her body) that indicate disease; for example, a complaint of feeling hot and having a hard time breathing*

■ **etiology:** *the science dealing with causes of disease. Etiology may also be defined as the study of all factors that might be involved in the development of a disease, including the susceptibility of the patient, the nature of the disease agent, and the way the patient's body is invaded by the agent*

■ **diagnose** *(verb):* identifying or recognizing a disease; done by scientific evaluation of the patient's signs and symptoms, physical assessment, history, laboratory tests, and investigative procedures. (How used: "What tests will you perform to diagnose the patient's disease?")

■ **diagnosis** *(noun):* the identification of a disease or condition; done after all of the evidence is evaluated and weighed. (How used: "The patient has a diagnosis of asthma.")

■ **treatment:** the care and management of a patient to prevent, minimize, or reverse a disease, disorder, or injury

■ **prognosis:** a prediction of the probable outcome of a disease based on the condition of the patient and the usual course of the disease as observed in similar situations

Epistaxis

Epistaxis has a clinical presentation of bleeding from the nose. Blood may be seen coming from either or both nostrils, or it can run down the back of the nasopharynx. Epistaxis is also called a *nosebleed*. (Review Figure 1–1 for the normal anatomy.)

Etiology

Epistaxis is primarily caused by picking of the nose, especially in children. Other causes include irritation of the mucous membrane from a nasogastric (feeding) tube, dry mucous membranes, trauma, hypertension, or clotting disorder.

Diagnosis

Bright red blood comes from the patient's nose. Pain is often associated with the bleeding.

Treatment

The patient should lean forward to let the blood flow out of the nostrils, breathe through the mouth, and not swallow the blood. Bleeding can usually be stopped within a few minutes by pinching the nostrils, putting a cotton ball in the nostril(s), or putting an ice-water compress over the nose. If the bleeding does not stop, a physician may have to cauterize (burn) the bleeding area or pack it with gauze.

Prognosis

The patient should recover completely from a nosebleed.

Upper Respiratory Tract Infection

An upper respiratory tract infection (URI) may involve headache, sinus drainage and runny nose, tearing eyes, sore throat, earache, hoarseness (laryngitis), and/or productive cough. (Review Figures 1–1 and 1–2 for the normal anatomy.) Children often have this problem; adults tend to have fewer episodes.

Clinical Presentation

The patient appears sick and often has a low-grade fever. Symptoms can relate to the nasal passage, throat, ears, and large airways. In some cases the infection spreads to all these areas, whereas other patients will have more isolated symptoms.

Etiology

Viral infections lead to most cases of URI. However, a bacterial infection can follow after the viral infection. Most people consider a URI to be a "common cold."

Diagnosis

A typical URI history relates to exposure to someone with a cold and development of symptoms related to an upper respiratory tract infection. The physician may rub a sterile swab in the patient's nasal passage or throat to check for a bacterial infection.

Treatment

The symptoms of a URI are treated with nasal decongestants, cough syrups, aspirin, ibuprofen, or acetaminophen for headache, drinking juices, and getting rest. There are no medications to kill the viruses that cause URIs. If a bacterial infection is proven, the physician may order an antibiotic.

Prognosis

A common cold from a virus runs its course in about a week. The patient should recover completely. However, some patients may suffer from another (secondary) bacterial infection. This can be a more serious problem.

Obstructive Sleep Apnea

Obstructive sleep apnea involves a patient stopping breathing for frequent, short periods of time while sleeping. During sleep, the patient's tongue and throat muscles relax and block the upper airway. (See Figure 1–1 for the normal upper airway anatomy.)

Clinical Presentation

The patient's spouse/bed partner complains of the patient's loud snoring, apnea periods, and daytime sleepiness. The physician will likely find various cardiopulmonary changes that result from repeated episodes of hypoxemia from sleep apnea.

Etiology

Many, but not necessarily all, of the following factors are seen in patients with obstructive sleep apnea: obesity, small jaw, large tonsils and adenoids, and small oral pharynx.

Diagnosis

The history of the patient's sleep pattern is important. It is usually given by the spouse/bed partner, as the patient is unaware of the breathing problems during sleep. The physician will examine the patient's upper airway and possibly take x-rays of the neck and/or chest. Pulmonary function tests and an electrocardiogram may be taken to check for lung or heart disease. Ideally, a sleep apnea study will be performed. This involves the patient being monitored and observed during a period of sleep to look for abnormal breathing patterns.

Treatment

Continuous positive airway pressure (CPAP) is often used when these patients sleep. The CPAP dilates the upper airway and pushes the tongue forward so that the airway stays open. In some cases surgery is performed to remove the tonsils and adenoids or enlarge the oral pharynx.

Prognosis

Patients who are properly diagnosed and treated for their sleep apnea will do very well. Untreated sleep apnea can result in pulmonary and cardiac disease, the result of repeated periods of hypoxemia when the patient does not breathe while sleeping.

▬▬ PULMONARY SYSTEM PROBLEMS: LOWER (SMALLER) AIRWAY

Small airways problems are usually serious. Reduction of air movement or complete blockage of air movement to the lungs will reduce the patient's oxygen level.

Asthma

Asthma is a respiratory disorder characterized by recurring attacks of severe difficulty in breathing (dyspnea) and normal breathing between episodes. Four airway problems are found in a patient having an asthma attack:

1. *Bronchospasm,* which is constriction of the muscles wrapped around the small airways.
2. **Inflammation** of the tissues in the airways.
3. Increased production of sticky mucus.
4. Sloughing off of the tissues in the airways.

A severe asthma attack that does not respond to treatment is called *status asthmaticus* and can be fatal. (See Figures 1–5, 1–6, and 1–7 to review normal anatomy.)

Clinical Presentation

Asthma has a clinical presentation of wheezing breath sounds, dyspnea, air trapping in the lungs, and hypoxemia.

Etiology

Many external and internal factors can trigger an asthma attack in someone who has **allergies.** Examples of external factors include, but are not limited to, inhaled house dust, animal dander, pollen, smoke, fumes, foods such as eggs, milk, nuts, and fish; and aerosols of cleaning agents. Examples of internal factors include emotional upset and airway infections.

■ *inflammation: the protective response of the tissues of the body to irritation or injury*

■ *allergies: acquired, hypersensitive reactions to normally harmless substances (allergens) found in nature. Examples of substances that cause allergies include house dust, pollen, and foods such as eggs. Upon first exposure to the allergen, the body becomes sensitive to it and creates antibodies to fight the allergen. The second and following exposures to the allergen cause the antibodies to fight against it, causing harm to the body in the process*

Diagnosis

The patient's history points to contact with an allergen that has triggered a previous asthma attack. Physical exam reveals air trapping, wheezing breath sounds, use of accessory muscles of breathing, dyspnea, and cyanosis. Pulmonary functions tests show decreased flow of air out of the lungs. Arterial blood gas analysis shows hypoxemia. In severe cases, the patient's carbon dioxide level is elevated and mechanical ventilation is required (see Chapter 3).

Treatment

Several different classes of medications are used to relax (dilate) the airway (bronchial) muscles. Collectively these medications are called *bronchodilators*. Usually the patient inhales the medicine directly into the lungs. See Figures 3-18 and 3-19 for examples of the devices. Sometimes the medication is given by an intravenous (IV) catheter. Patients who do not respond to these airway relaxation medications are said to have *status asthmaticus* and require supported breathing on a mechanical ventilator. Patient education is important so that the patient learns how to avoid allergens and prevent a future asthma attack.

Prognosis

Patients who avoid allergens and take their medications can have a normal life. Between asthma episodes, their lungs return to normal. However, some patients have reduced lung function even though they take their medications. About 5,000 people die each year in the United States from asthma. Asthma is often referred to as a **chronic obstructive pulmonary disease (COPD).**

■ *chronic obstructive pulmonary disease (COPD): a progressive and irreversible condition characterized by decreased airflow on expiration, overinflated lungs, and shortness of breath; COPD includes asthma, chronic bronchitis, and emphysema*

Bronchitis

Bronchitis is an airway disease in which the mucous membranes of the tracheobronchial tree are inflamed. (See Figures 1–5, 1–6, and 1–7 to review normal anatomy.) Acute bronchitis is seen in patients who have an upper airway viral infection that spreads to the lower airways. *Chronic bronchitis* is defined as a productive cough for at least three consecutive months in the last two consecutive years.

Clinical Presentation

Bronchitis patients have a productive cough with infected secretions, fever, and discomfort in the airways or chest muscles from coughing.

Etiology

Acute bronchitis is usually caused by a viral or bacterial upper airway infection that spreads to the lower airways. It is seen frequently in children after a head cold or other childhood infection. Chronic bronchitis is a more serious problem that is caused by cigarette smoking, chronic bacterial infection of the airways, or cystic fibrosis (see discussion later in this chapter). Chronic bronchitis is often considered a chronic obstructive pulmonary disease.

Diagnosis

The patient reports a productive cough that is associated with an airway infection. A sputum sample may be taken to identify the type of organism causing the infection. Breath sounds will reveal secretions in the airways. The patient will often have a high fever and appear sick. Pulmonary function tests are done with patients who have chronic bronchitis to determine the extent of lung damage.

Treatment

Avoid any inhaled irritants. If the patient smokes, he or she must be told to stop. An antibiotic may be ordered to fight off the infection. An expectorant may be given to make the secretions easier to cough out.

Prognosis

Most people recover completely from a case of acute bronchitis within a week or two. However, the infection may develop into pneumonia, which could have serious consequences. People with chronic bronchitis from smoking may have done serious damage to their airways and lungs. Depending on how damaged the airways and lungs are, the patient may have exercise and other limits.

Bronchogenic Carcinoma

Bronchogenic carcinoma is cancer of the airways and/or the lung(s). The cancer often starts in an airway and then penetrates into lung tissue.

Clinical Presentation

Clinical presentation of bronchogenic carcinoma often includes a cough productive of blood, shortness of breath, recent significant loss of weight, fatigue, and cancer found in another part of the body.

Etiology

Most cases of lung cancer are caused by cigarette smoking. Other causes of lung cancer include exposure to inhaled asbestos, uranium, radon gas, or toxic fumes.

Diagnosis

The patient will have a history of smoking or exposure to another cancer-causing agent. He or she will report recent loss of weight, coughing up bloody sputum, fatigue, and/or shortness of breath. A chest x-ray or bronchoscopy exam will often find a lung tumor. (Chest x-ray and bronchoscopy are discussed in Chapter 3.)

Treatment

If the tumor is isolated in a particular segment or lobe of the lung, it may be surgically removed. (See Figure 1–8 for lung anatomy.) If surgery cannot be done, the patient may be treated by **radiation** to the lung or **chemotherapy.**

■ *radiation:* the use of radioactive materials to destroy cancer cells by making them unable to reproduce

■ *chemotherapy:* the use of chemicals to destroy cancer cells by making them unable to reproduce

Prognosis

Most patients do not survive a lung cancer or cancer that has spread from the lung to other parts of the body. The five-year survival rate is about 10%.

Cystic Fibrosis

Cystic fibrosis (CF) is an inherited genetic defect that prevents or slows down the movement of water into the mucous membranes of the body. This causes the patient to have very thick secretions that are difficult to cough out. Cystic fibrosis is first seen in young children.

Clinical Presentation

Children with cystic fibrosis present with chronic bronchitis, poor weight gain, and difficult, foul-smelling bowel movements.

Etiology

Cystic fibrosis is a genetic defect. It decreases the ability of water to enter the mucous membranes of the lungs, intestines, and reproductive tracts of both males and females.

Diagnosis

The parents usually bring the infant to the physician because of a lung infection or failure to grow. Physical exam and history point out frequent lung infections, difficult bowel movements, and malnutrition despite being well fed. Specific laboratory tests can show that the child has cystic fibrosis. A history of the parents usually reveals that they both have had blood relatives with cystic fibrosis.

Treatment

The patient will be given a special diet, vitamins, and medications to help him or her digest and absorb food better. Antibiotics are given to treat the pulmonary infections that frequently affect these children. Expectorants are given to keep the mucus easy to cough out. Postural drainage therapy (discussed in Chapter 3) is done to drain mucus from the lungs.

Prognosis

Sadly, most of these children die of pulmonary infections and complications before they reach adulthood. With good treatment, however, some are now living into their twenties and thirties.

■■■ PULMONARY SYSTEM PROBLEMS: LUNGS

All lung problems are serious. Diseases that affect the lungs will reduce the amount of oxygen that can get to the blood to go to the body. If the oxygen level falls too low, it can be fatal.

Atelectasis

Atelectasis is the collapse of alveoli so that they are airless. It may affect individual alveoli in different areas of the lungs, a whole segment, or a whole lobe.

Clinical Presentation

Clinical presentation of atelectasis includes diminished or absent breath sounds over the affected area(s) of the lung(s), shift of the mediastinum to the affected side, dyspnea, and low-grade fever. The patient may also have an increased respiratory rate, increased heart rate, and hypoxemia.

Etiology

Postoperative atelectasis is the result of patients not taking deep breaths because of pain at the surgical site. This is especially a problem when the patient has had thoracic or abdominal surgery. Other conditions such as fluid in the pleural space (see Figure 1–12) or a lung tumor can also cause atelectasis.

Diagnosis

Physical exam will reveal diminished or absent breath sounds over areas of atelectasis. If the collapsed area is large enough, the lung will shift toward that side. This results in a mediastinal shift toward the area of lung collapse as well.

Treatment

If the patient recently had surgery, it is important to get him or her up and out of bed as soon as possible. Additionally, have the patient take deep breaths and cough and perform a treatment called incentive spirometry to open up the areas of atelectasis. (These treatments are discussed in Chapter 3.) If there is fluid in the pleural space, it should be removed. The patient with lung cancer will be treated for this more serious condition.

Prognosis

A patient with simple postoperative atelectasis should recover completely. However, if the patient's lungs do not reexpand, he or she will be at risk of getting pneumonia. This could be a very serious complication, as discussed later in this chapter. The prognosis for a patient with atelectasis secondary to pleural fluid buildup or lung cancer depends on the prognosis for the original problem.

Acute Respiratory Distress Syndrome

Acute respiratory distress syndrome (ARDS) is a very serious problem that occurs when the alveolar-capillary membrane is damaged and fluid from the pulmonary capillaries leaks into the alveoli. (See Figure 1–9 for normal anatomy.) (Note: Some references call this disease *adult* respiratory distress syndrome.)

Clinical Presentation

The clinical presentation for ARDS is a patient with very stiff, wet lungs; extreme dyspnea, rapid breathing and heart rate, and severe hypoxemia.

Etiology

ARDS is not an original disease. Rather, it is preceded—and caused—by some other problem that results in damage to the alveolar-capillary membrane. Examples of problems with the pulmonary capillary bed include blood infection (septicemia), pancreatitis (inflammation of the pancreas), and pulmonary embolism of fat. Examples of problems with the alveoli include inhalation of toxic chemicals, pneumonia, and aspiration (inhalation) of stomach contents.

Diagnosis

The patient will have had a previous problem, such as one of those listed earlier, that has led to lung damage. A chest x-ray will show fluid leakage into most areas of both lungs. Blood gas results will show severe hypoxemia even when the patient is receiving supplemental oxygen.

Treatment

The patient will almost always be mechanically ventilated with up to 100% oxygen. This is done to support the patient's breathing and prevent death from hypoxemia. The underlying condition must be treated so that the lung damage does not continue. The patient must also be medically supported in any other way that is needed.

Prognosis

Because ARDS causes serious damage to the alveolar-capillary membrane, the patient's ability to get oxygen into the blood is badly hampered. Approximately 50% of all patients who develop ARDS die from it or complications from the original disease.

Emphysema

Emphysema is dilation and destruction of alveoli and the capillary bed that surrounds them. Emphysema is often considered a chronic obstructive pulmonary disease.

Clinical Presentation

Patients with emphysema present with enlarged chest (so-called *barrel chest*), diminished breath sounds, flat diaphragm, and shortness of breath. Emphysema patients are usually hypoxemic and have an increased carbon dioxide level; many also have some degree of heart failure.

Etiology

Smoking tobacco is the leading cause of emphysema. Other causes include exposure to inhaled pollution and toxic fumes. Rarely, some patients are seen who have an inherited genetic defect that leads to emphysema.

Diagnosis

Most patients have a history of smoking or industrial contact with toxic fumes. If a patient is suspected of having genetic emphysema, the genetic defect is tested for. A pulmonary function test is performed to measure the patient's lung volumes and flow of air into and out of the lungs. A chest x-ray will show the lungs to be overinflated and the diaphragm flattened. Heart studies are also usually performed.

Treatment

Medication is available to help slow down the deterioration of the lungs in patients who have emphysema from a genetic defect. Unfortunately, the medication does not restore the lungs to their normal state. Patients who have lung disease from smoking or other inhaled toxins are told to stop smoking or avoid the toxin exposure. This will prevent further damage. Again, unfortunately, nothing can be done to restore lung function. The patient is supported so that he or she can have as good a life as possible. Supplemental oxygen is often needed. The oxygen may be required continuously, even at home.

Prognosis

Many patients with emphysema live for many years, although with a diminished quality of life. Death may be from lung or heart failure.

Pneumonia

Pneumonia is an infection of the lungs, including the alveoli and smallest airways. It is caused by the inhalation of microscopic organisms. Pneumonia can affect segment(s) or lobe(s) of one or both lungs. Many times a patient with pneumonia will also have bronchitis. When the infecting organism attacks the lung, the alveoli fill with fluid, live and dead organisms, and live and dead leukocytes. If the infection is widespread in both lungs, the hypoxemia can be quite severe. (See Figures 1–8 and 1–9 for normal anatomy.)

Clinical Presentation

The patient with pneumonia will present with a high fever, cough productive of mucus, shortness of breath, fast breathing and heart rates, and hypoxemia.

Etiology

Many different types of inhaled viruses, bacteria, and fungi can cause pneumonia and/or bronchitis.

Diagnosis

The patient's history may include a high fever, productive cough, and difficulty breathing. Often an upper respiratory tract infection precedes the chest problem. A sputum sample is obtained so that the laboratory can identify what microbe is causing the infection.

Treatment

If the infectious organism is a bacterium or fungus, an appropriate antibiotic is given to kill it. Unfortunately, no medications are available to kill viruses. All patients must rest, eat well, and let their bodies heal. Often supplemental oxygen is needed. Mechanical ventilation may also be required.

Prognosis

Patients with viral infections usually heal completely in a few weeks. Most patients with a bacterial or fungal infection who were healthy before the infection, and who are promptly given the right antibiotic, will heal completely within a few weeks. However, some patients delay seeing a doctor until the infection has progressed too far. They, and other patients who were not healthy before becoming infected, may die of the pulmonary infection. The very young, the very old, and those with weakened immune systems are most likely to die from pneumonia.

Pulmonary Edema

Pulmonary edema is fluid that has leaked from the pulmonary capillary bed into the alveoli. In severe cases the fluid may fill the airways and hamper effective breathing.

Clinical Presentation

The patient will be very short of breath, have rapid breathing and heart rates, and low blood pressure. The patient will usually show hypoxemia.

Etiology

Edema fluid can leak into alveoli when the alveolar-capillary membrane is damaged, as in acute respiratory distress syndrome (ARDS). Also, heart failure can result in fluid backing up into the pulmonary circulation and then leaking into the alveoli.

Diagnosis

A chest x-ray is taken to find the extent of the pulmonary edema and to look at the size of the heart. A large heart is usually seen with heart failure but not with ARDS. The patient's history is also important because it will usually indicate a preceding episode of heart failure or an injury or illness that would lead to ARDS.

Treatment

The treatment depends on the original cause of the pulmonary edema. This original problem must be treated. If the patient has heart failure, the heart weakness must be treated with heart-strengthening medications. If the patient has too much fluid in his or her system, a medication is given to make the kidneys put out more urine. The patient may need to be placed on a mechanical ventilator with supplemental oxygen to support his or her breathing.

Prognosis

The patient's prognosis depends on the underlying problem and how much pulmonary edema is present. Patients with heart failure and the resulting pulmonary edema may be severely hypoxic and can die.

Pulmonary Fibrosis

Pulmonary fibrosis is the formation of scar tissue in the lungs.

Clinical Presentation

The patient with this problem will present clinically with stiff lungs, rapid respiratory rate, small tidal volume, and hypoxemia.

Etiology

Chronic, long-term exposure to inhaled inorganic dust or small airborne particles commonly causes pulmonary fibrosis.

Diagnosis

A pulmonary function test will reveal that all lung volumes and capacities are small. A chest x-ray will show small lungs with increased lung markings from scar tissue. The patient's history will usually reveal an earlier exposure to inhaled asbestos, silica, or coal dust.

Treatment

The patient must avoid all future contact with dust or smoke. There is no cure for the pulmonary fibrosis, so it is important that the patient be careful not to cause further injury. Supplemental oxygen may be needed so that the patient can remain active.

Prognosis

Many patients can live for a prolonged time with stable pulmonary fibrosis.

▬▬ THORAX AND ABDOMEN

The thorax and abdomen support and protect the lungs and heart. Additionally, the contraction of muscles there pulls air into the lungs for breathing. Injury to the thorax or abdomen can impair the patient's ability to breathe.

Trauma

Trauma is physical injury caused by a violent or disruptive action. Major trauma to the chest wall, or in some cases the abdomen, can interfere with the ability to breathe. This is especially true when a person has multiple broken ribs. A *flail chest* is when a person has three or more adjacent ribs broken in two or more places. The flail chest area does not move in coordination with the rest of the chest wall during breathing. If a lung is punctured, the patient will have a **pneumothorax.** Air will be found inside the pleural space and it will cause the lung to collapse.

■ *pneumothorax: a collection of air or gas in the pleural space that causes the lung to collapse. When the air is under pressure, there is said to be a* tension pneumothorax; *this causes the lungs, heart, and mediastinal structures to shift to the opposite side*

Clinical Presentation

The patient with chest trauma will have an obvious injury. The following may be found: tissue injury, blood, pain at the injury site, difficult breathing, unstable chest wall, low blood pressure from loss of blood, and hypoxemia. (See Figures 1–11 and 1–12 for normal anatomy.)

Etiology

A serious injury can occur from an automobile accident, industrial accident, fight, gunshot, stabbing, fall from height, and the like.

Diagnosis

The patient will have a history of injury. A physical exam will find an injured chest wall or abdomen. A chest x-ray will be taken to look for broken ribs, punctured lung, or other internal injury.

Treatment

Treatment will depend on the nature of the injury. The patient who is too injured to effectively breathe spontaneously will be placed on a mechanical ventilator. If a lung has been punctured, the air must be removed from the pleural space so that the lung can reexpand. (The procedures called *thoracentesis* and *closed-chest drainage* to remove the air are discussed in Chapter 3.)

Prognosis

If the patient is promptly treated for the injury, the chance of recovery is good. However, some injuries are so extensive, and blood loss so great, that the patient may die at the scene of the injury or after transportation to a hospital.

■■■ DISEASE OF THE MUSCLES OF BREATHING

At least two types of diseases affect the proper functioning of the muscles of breathing. *Muscular dystrophy (MD)* is a group of inherited diseases that cause a progressive **atrophy** of symmetric groups of skeletal muscles. *Myasthenia gravis* is a disease of the junction of the nerves and skeletal muscles (myoneural junction) that results in weakness and fatigue.

■ *atrophy: a wasting or decrease of size or function of a part of the body because of disease or other influences. Skeletal muscles undergo atrophy when nerve damage or disease prevents their being exercised*

Clinical Presentation

When the breathing muscles do not function normally, the patient may experience problems ranging from difficulty in taking a deep breath and coughing, to easy fatigue with exercise, to complete lack of ability to breathe. The patient's breathing rate may be fast in an attempt to compensate for shallow tidal volume breathing.

Etiology

Muscular dystrophy is a genetic defect in the patient's metabolism that affects muscle function. Myasthenia gravis is an imbalance in the chemicals that make the myoneural junction work properly.

Diagnosis

The diagnosis for muscular dystrophy is made by genetic testing, muscle biopsy, and electrical stimulation of affected muscles. Myasthenia gravis is diagnosed by a test that corrects the chemical imbalance found at the myoneural junction and causes increased muscle strength.

Treatment

There is no direct treatment for muscular dystrophy. The patient is aided by braces to support the affected limbs. Myasthenia gravis patients can be treated with medications that restore the normal balance of chemicals at the myoneural junction.

Prognosis

Patients with muscular dystrophy can live for many years with the disease. However, death is usually caused by respiratory failure. Myasthenia gravis patients can usually lead fairly normal lives, but may still have problems with fatigue if they try to do too much.

■■■ HEART AND CIRCULATORY SYSTEM PROBLEMS

Blood must be able to circulate through the vessels of the heart muscle to bring it oxygen, like any other part of the body. Blood must be able to flow through the lungs' circulatory system for oxygen and carbon dioxide to be exchanged. A blockage of any major vessel in the heart or lungs is very serious—death can result.

Heart Disease

Heart disease is a general term that refers to any pathological condition of the heart. It is important to understand that four different types of problems can affect the heart. First, a patient can have coronary artery disease, which is a narrowing of one or more of the coronary arteries by the buildup of fatty deposits (*atherosclerosis*). Second, a patient can have damage or a defect in one or more of the heart valves. Third, a patient can have heart failure. This is a condition in which the weakened heart cannot pump enough blood to meet the needs of the body. Congestive heart failure is a condition in which a weakened heart exists along with an increase in the amount of fluid in the body. Fourth, the patient can have a myocardial infarction (heart attack). This occurs when the complete blockage of a coronary artery prevents blood from reaching a part of the heart muscle so that the affected muscle dies.

Clinical Presentation

Common symptoms include fast heart rate, low blood pressure, edema in the feet and lungs, fatigue, shortness of breath, and pain in the chest or radiated down the left arm (*angina*). Not all patients will have all of these symptoms.

Etiology

Coronary artery disease is caused by high blood cholesterol, smoking, obesity, diabetes, high blood pressure, and physical inactivity. Atherosclerosis can decrease the heart's blood supply so much that heart failure develops. Complete blockage of the coronary artery by atherosclerosis or a blood clot will cause a myocardial infarction. Heart valve problems can result from the valve not developing properly in the fetus or from an infection of the heart valve.

Diagnosis

A physical exam will reveal fast heart rate, low blood pressure, abnormal heart sounds, and/or fluid buildup in the feet and lungs. An electrocardiogram will show abnormal heart rate and rhythm. Arterial blood gases will show hypoxemia. The blood of a patient with a myocardial infarction will have specific chemical markers showing heart damage. Special heart tests can be done that involve passing a long catheter into the heart or coronary arteries and injecting dye to check on proper functioning. (See Figures 1–17 and 1–20 for normal anatomy.)

Treatment

Coronary artery disease is prevented by changing the patient's lifestyle so that he or she eats more sensibly, stops smoking, loses weight, and exercises. In some cases the clogged interior of a coronary artery is opened up by a procedure called *angioplasty*. In this procedure a catheter is placed into the artery and the fatty deposits are flattened out or removed. This is sometimes also done to dilate the artery to prevent a myocardial infarction. If a blood clot is suspected of causing a myocardial infarction, a clot-dissolving drug will probably be given. Sometimes a patient needs to have open heart surgery to have a coronary artery bypass graft (CABG) placed around the narrowed or blocked artery. Open heart surgery is often performed to repair or replace a defective heart valve. A patient with heart failure is treated with medications to strengthen the heart and other medications to make the kidneys put out more urine, as well as the other treatments for coronary artery disease. Supplemental oxygen is given as needed. Many times a patient with heart disease of any kind will require breathing support on a mechanical ventilator. Cardiopulmonary resuscitation (CPR) may have to be performed.

Prognosis

Many patients who receive prompt care for their heart disease can have it corrected and lead fairly normal lives. However, some problems, like myocardial infarction, are so severe that the patient dies when it happens or shortly thereafter.

Pulmonary Embolism

Pulmonary embolism means that a thrombus (blood clot) or other particulate matter has entered the circulatory system and become lodged in a branch of the pulmonary artery. (See Figure 1–21 for normal anatomy.)

Clinical Presentation

The patient will feel sudden shortness of breath. This may be accompanied by chest pain or coughing up of blood. Arterial blood gas values will show hypoxemia.

Etiology

The following things can become a pulmonary embolism: blood clot from a leg vein, fat or marrow from a broken bone, tumor fragment, amniotic fluid, or air bubble from a venous catheter.

Diagnosis

A special pulmonary function test called a ventilation-perfusion (V/Q) scan will be performed. This test involves the patient inhaling a radioactive gas and having a radioactive substance injected into his or her venous system. The results will show that pulmonary artery blood flow is cut off or reduced to one or more parts of the lung(s).

Treatment

Supplemental oxygen is given to correct any hypoxemia. If a blood clot is suspected, a clot-dissolving drug will probably be given. If the patient is at risk of having more blood clots in the legs, a medication will be given to slow down the clotting process (an anticoagulant or so-called "blood thinner"). Sometimes a patient will require support on a mechanical ventilator.

Prognosis

Patients with small pulmonary emboli should recover completely. A massive pulmonary embolism that completely blocks blood flow to one or both lungs can result in death.

▓▓▓ CONTROL OF BREATHING PROBLEMS

The brain and nervous system must be operating normally to send signals to the muscles that control breathing. A variety of diseases can affect the brain, spinal cord, and other nerves so that breathing is impaired. Obviously, this can be life-threatening.

Medication Overdose

At least three different types of medications affect the brain's respiratory center and can depress a patient's breathing. Sedatives are designed to relax a person or put him or her to sleep. These include antianxiety medications (like Valium) and sleeping pills. When used properly, they will not cause any breathing problems. However, sometimes a person accidentally or purposefully takes an overdose. Muscle relaxants are designed to control muscle spasms or relieve back muscle pain. Again, sometimes a person accidentally or purposefully takes an overdose. Powerful pain-relieving agents (like morphine) directly affect the brain so that the patient feels less pain. Sometimes a hospitalized patient is accidentally given too much and his or her breathing center is affected—the patient's breathing will slow down or stop altogether.

Clinical Presentation

A patient who has received too much of any of these medications will be unconscious and will have either a slow respiratory rate and shallow breathing or have completely stopped breathing (apnea). The blood pressure will be low and the heart rate will probably be low.

Etiology

Cause is accidental or intentional overdose of a sedative, muscle relaxant, or pain-relieving medication. If taken in a large enough amount, any of these medications will adversely affect the respiratory center of the brain. (See Figure 1–15, for normal anatomy.)

Diagnosis

The medication bottle may be found with the patient, or street-drug equipment may be found. A blood sample from the patient will identify the overdose medication.

Treatment

The patient's airway must be secured with a breathing tube. Mechanical ventilation will be needed. The patient's stomach will be pumped out to remove any remaining medication. If an antidote to the overdose medication is available, it will be given. For example, Valium and morphine have direct antidotes.

Prognosis

If the patient has completely stopped breathing for more than a few minutes, he or she will have suffered irreversible damage to the brain from hypoxemia. Sadly, this is often the case. If the patient did not stop breathing or normal breathing is quickly restored, the patient will probably recover completely.

Brain Injury

The brain can be injured by a stroke (cerebrovascular accident or CVA), brain tumor, or direct trauma. These events, which can cause paralysis, inability to speak, and other problems, may also cause the respiratory center of the brain to fail to send out normal signals for breathing.

Clinical Presentation

The patient may have an abnormal breathing pattern with variable respiratory rate, tidal volume, and/or inspiratory to expiratory timing. Additionally, the patient may be unable to swallow or protect the airway and be prone to the inhalation (aspiration) of food and liquids. Aspiration can obstruct the airways and lead to hypoxemia and/or pneumonia.

Etiology

A stroke can be caused by a blood clot in one of the brain's arteries. Also, a brain artery can rupture, causing bleeding in the brain. A brain tumor will compress normal brain tissue. Direct trauma can be from a car accident, fall from height, or being struck by a heavy object or bullet.

Diagnosis

The patient's history will reveal what happened to the patient to affect his or her brain. A series of special head and brain x-rays may show the problem. Observation will determine the type of abnormal breathing pattern the patient has.

Treatment

If the patient has a blood clot, a clot-dissolving medication will probably be given. Surgery may be performed to remove a brain tumor or correct an injury. The patient's breathing will be supported on a mechanical ventilator if necessary.

Prognosis

The prognosis will vary considerably based on how severely the brain is injured. Some patients will recover most of their bodily functions, including breathing. Others will live but suffer major, permanent impairment. Unfortunately, others will die due to failure of the medulla and pons areas of the brain to regulate breathing, blood pressure, and heart rate.

Nervous System Injury or Disease

Injuries or diseases that affect the spinal cord or peripheral nerves to the respiratory muscles can prevent nerve signals from the brain from reaching the muscles. When this happens, different sets of muscles may be unable to function, even though others may work normally. The patient may be able to have a normal tidal volume breath but be unable to take in a deep breath. *Guillain-Barré syndrome* is a disease that damages the covering of the nerves (myelin sheath). This prevents the nerve signal from reaching the nerves throughout the body. Trauma to the spinal cord can result in partial or complete **paralysis.** This can affect not only the legs and arms but also the breathing muscles. A spinal cord injury that is below the fourth or fifth cervical (neck) vertebra will cause paralysis to the body. However, the phrenic nerves will still send signals to the diaphragm for tidal volume breathing. A spinal cord injury that is above the

■ *paralysis: the loss of muscle function, sensation, or both. Paralysis may be further defined by location in the body, such as right side, left side, legs, and so on*

fourth cervical vertebra will result in injury to the phrenic nerves. They will not operate to send signals to the diaphragm and the patient will be completely unable to breathe. (See Figure 1–13 for normal anatomy.)

Clinical Presentation

The patient with Guillain-Barré syndrome will have gradual weakness and then paralysis starting at the feet and hands and moving to the body. After a period of total paralysis, the nerves will regrow. The patient will then be able to breathe again and the arms and legs will regain movement. A patient with a spinal cord injury will have suffered some traumatic event and may have other injuries as well. Paralysis will be present in the affected areas.

Etiology

Guillain-Barré syndrome is usually preceded by a viral infection. For unknown reasons, the body makes antibodies that invade and damage the myelin sheath. As stated earlier, a spinal cord injury is caused by some traumatic event.

Diagnosis

The patient with Guillain-Barré syndrome will have a history of a viral infection. A blood sample will show the presence of antibodies. The pattern of paralysis starting at the extremities and moving to the body is seen only with this disease. The spinal cord trauma patient will have a history of injury and resulting paralysis.

Treatment

The patient with Guillain-Barré syndrome will need to be supported on a mechanical ventilator until the nerves begin to function again. He or she can then be taken off the machine. The patient must continue to be fed and cared for until the disease runs its course. The patient with a spinal cord injury must be supported as needed. He or she may require temporary or permanent breathing support on a mechanical ventilator. Physical therapy services may be used to help the patient learn how to care for himself or herself within the limits of the paralysis. Support equipment and services such as wheelchairs and household aides will make activities of daily living easier.

Prognosis

Most Guillain-Barré syndrome patients recover completely within a few months. Unfortunately, spinal cord injury patients cannot expect any recovery from the paralysis.

▰▰▰ BLOOD PROBLEMS

As you know, the blood carries oxygen and carbon dioxide throughout the body. Conditions that reduce the number of erythrocytes (red blood cells) or prevent their functioning will reduce the patient's oxygen supply. If the restriction is severe enough, the patient can die.

Carbon Monoxide Poisoning

Carbon monoxide (CO) is a colorless, odorless, tasteless gas that binds (chemically attaches) to erythrocytes in the same manner as oxygen does. However, carbon monoxide has a much higher binding strength than oxygen and will displace it from erythrocytes. This prevents the blood from carrying oxygen and causes severe hypoxemia.

Clinical Presentation

Conscious patients complain of headache, drowsiness, nausea, and/or confusion. If the patient's carbon monoxide level is high enough, he or she will be unconscious and may have an abnormal cardiac rhythm.

Etiology

The most common source of carbon monoxide poisoning is inhalation of exhaust fumes from an automobile. Other common sources of CO include smoke from a house fire and a malfunctioning furnace that releases the gas into the house.

Diagnosis

History will include exposure to car exhaust fumes or another carbon monoxide source. An arterial blood gas sample will reveal an increased level of carbon monoxide.

Treatment

Remove the patient from the source of the carbon monoxide. Give the patient 100% oxygen to treat the hypoxemia. Support the patient's heart and lung function as needed until he or she has a normal, safe carbon monoxide level.

Prognosis

Patients who have inhaled a high level of carbon monoxide at the scene of a house fire or other source are often found dead. If the patient's carbon monoxide level is not immediately fatal, and he or she is treated with oxygen at the hospital, recovery can be expected. However, some patients will survive but suffer brain damage.

Anemia

Anemia is a decrease below normal in the number or volume of erythrocytes (red blood cells) or in the quantity of hemoglobin in the blood. Because of the low number of erythrocytes, the patient cannot carry the normal amount of oxygen in the blood.

Clinical Presentation

Patients with mild anemia will complain of becoming easily tired. Patients with severe anemia will complain of shortness of breath and have a rapid heart rate.

Etiology

Anemia is the result of either a loss of blood or the inability of the body to make enough new erythrocytes. Loss of blood can be from an injury, surgery, or internal bleeding from an ulcer or cancer. Poor diet or abnormal bone marrow can result in low production of erythrocytes.

Treatment

Severe anemia is treated by giving the patient blood that matches his or her own (a transfusion). Poor diet can be corrected by eating the right types and quantities of food containing iron. Bone marrow problems are more difficult to treat.

Prognosis

Severe, sudden anemia from bleeding can be fatal. If the bleeding is stopped and new blood is given, the patient may recover completely.

REVIEW QUESTIONS

Multiple Choice Questions

1. Your patient is being evaluated for obstructive sleep apnea. While observing him, you notice that he has gone 20 seconds without breathing. He then awakens and breathes normally. What would you do?
   a. Wake him up and do not let him go back to sleep.
   b. Report your observations to the registered nurse or respiratory care practitioner.
   c. Put an oxygen mask on him.
   d. Put a CPAP mask on him.

2. The prognosis for a patient with bronchogenic carcinoma is:
   a. Good; complete recovery is expected.
   b. Fair; most patients recover completely.
   c. Guarded; about half of the patients recover.
   d. Poor; few patients recover.

3. Which of the following diseases is inherited?
   a. Cystic fibrosis
   b. Acute respiratory distress syndrome
   c. Pulmonary fibrosis
   d. Guillain-Barré syndrome

4. Coronary artery disease is caused by all of the following *except:*
   a. Caucasian race.
   b. Obesity.
   c. Smoking.
   d. Diabetes.

5. The most common cause of a pulmonary embolism is:
   a. Air bubble.
   b. Bone marrow.
   c. Blood clot.
   d. Tumor fragment.

6. All of the following medications can depress breathing *except:*
   a. Sleeping pills.
   b. Pain-relieving medications.
   c. Muscle-relaxing medications.
   d. Antibiotics.

7. How is carbon monoxide poisoning treated?
   a. Giving carbon dioxide.
   b. Giving 100% oxygen.
   c. Giving 21% oxygen.
   d. Giving a blood transfusion.

8. A patient with a spinal cord injury can expect:
   a. Complete recovery within one to two months.
   b. Partial recovery within one to two months.
   c. Permanent paralysis of the affected area.

9. A myocardial infarction:
   a. Is the same thing as a stroke.
   b. Is the same thing as a heart attack.
   c. Is a blood clot in the lung.
   d. Is caused by so-called blood-thinning medications.

10. All of the following are referred to as chronic obstructive pulmonary diseases (COPD) *except:*
    a. Chronic bronchitis.
    b. Emphysema.
    c. Atelectasis.
    d. Asthma.

11. Inhaled microorganisms that reach the alveoli can cause:
    a. Pneumonia.
    b. Epistaxis.
    c. Pneumothorax.
    d. Pulmonary fibrosis.

12. All of the following problems are found in a patient with asthma *except:*
    a. Increased mucus production.
    b. Edema of the mucous membranes of the airways.
    c. Bronchospasm.
    d. Bleeding in the airways.

Introduction to Respiratory Care Procedures

After reading this chapter, you will be able to:

Identify the role of the respiratory care practitioner in each of the covered diagnostic tests and treatment procedures.

Identify the possible role(s) of the patient care technician in each of the covered diagnostic tests and treatment procedures.

Identify the purpose(s) of the covered diagnostic tests and treatment procedures.

OVERVIEW

This final chapter is designed to help you understand the role of the respiratory care profession and some common diagnostic tests and treatments for patients with cardiopulmonary diseases. It would be helpful for you to become familiar with these tests and treatments because you will likely see them being done with patients. However, only the most important features are presented. Other aspects of the tests and treatments are not presented, because of their complexity. Additionally, some diagnostic tests and treatments are not presented at all because it is less likely that you will see them or be involved in caring for patients receiving them.

Competency checkoff lists are provided in the Appendix for a number of procedures that may be used in the care of patients with lung or heart conditions. Depending on your place of work, you as a patient care technician (PCT) may be expected to perform some or all of these procedures. It is up to your employer to determine which, if any, of these procedures you may perform. It is also your employer's responsibility to provide additional training to you so that you are competent on those procedures that they expect you to perform.

Never attempt to perform any patient care procedure that you have not been trained for. Always get help from a respiratory care practitioner (RCP) or **registered nurse (RN)** if you have trouble with any treatment or test.

THE RESPIRATORY CARE PROFESSION

The national professional organization for respiratory care is the American Association for Respiratory Care (AARC). All 50 states have chapters, in addition to three international ones. The AARC and the state chapters are involved in monitoring state and national health care legislation, encouraging smoking cessation, and other health care issues. The AARC has released this definition of *respiratory care:*

Respiratory Care is a life-supporting, life-enhancing health care profession practiced under qualified medical direction. Medical direction means that the practice of respiratory care is provided under a medical director. Respiratory care services provided to patients with disorders of the cardiopulmonary system include: diagnostic testing, therapeutics, monitoring, and rehabilitation. Patient, family, and public education are central to the

■ **Key Concept:**
*Simply reading this text does **not** qualify you to perform the procedures presented here or any other patient care procedures. If, at any time, you observe a patient problem that could be dangerous, contact your supervisor immediately!* ■

■ *registered nurse (RN):*
a professional nurse who has completed a course of study at a state-approved school of nursing and passed the National Council Licensure Examination

mission of the profession. Respiratory care services are provided in all health care facilities and in the home.

The respiratory care profession has two levels of practitioner. Respiratory therapy technicians must graduate from a 12- to 18-month post-secondary or hospital-based program. Graduates receive a certificate and can take a national credentialing examination. Upon passing the examination they are awarded the credential of *Certified Respiratory Therapy Technician* (CRTT). Respiratory therapists usually graduate from either a two-year associate's degree or a four-year bachelor's degree program. They may earn the CRTT credential and take further examinations to earn the *Registered Respiratory Therapist* (RRT) credential.

The general term *respiratory care practitioner (RCP)* is often used to include both levels of respiratory care professional. Many states have included the RCP term in their legislation governing the practice of respiratory care. RCP is used in this chapter to refer to any respiratory care professional.

THE ATMOSPHERE

■ **atmosphere:** *gases surrounding the earth or any planet*

■ **nitrogen:** *a gaseous element that makes up 78% of the earth's atmosphere. It plays no part in ventilation or respiration. Its compounds are essential for life and are found in proteins and nucleic acids*

■ **helium:** *a gas that is the second lightest element known (after hydrogen)*

■ **ozone:** *a gas formed from the combination of three oxygen atoms. A layer of ozone surrounds the earth at an altitude of 20 to 30 miles and protects the earth from excessive ultraviolet radiation from the sun. When ozone is found close to the earth, it is considered to be a form of air pollution and is an airway irritant*

Earth's **atmosphere** extends from sea level to a height of about 30 miles. Our atmosphere is made up primarily of just two gases: nitrogen and oxygen. **Nitrogen** (N_2) makes up 78% of our atmosphere. Despite its being the main gas of our planet, nitrogen gas does not interact in any way with people or other animals. We breathe it in and out constantly without its having any benefit or doing any harm to us. Oxygen (O_2) makes up almost 21% of our atmosphere. As you know, oxygen is vital for the body's metabolism. The last 1% of earth's atmosphere is made up of small amounts of a variety of other gases, such as carbon dioxide, **helium, ozone,** and others. All of these gases are equally mixed throughout the atmosphere.

Water vapor is also found in the atmosphere but is not counted as one of the main gases. Water vapor is liquid water that has been warmed and turned to a gas. When water vapor cools, clouds are formed. Further cooling can cause rain (or snow if the temperature is below freezing). The amount of water vapor in the air varies considerably based on local open water and weather conditions.

Earth's gravity keeps the atmosphere here and prevents it from going off into space. Because of gravity, the air is more tightly packed at the earth's surface and becomes more loosely packed the higher you go. This is why people have more difficulty breathing on top of mountains (like Denver, Colorado) and high-flying airplanes must have their cabins pressurized.

CAUSES OF HYPOXEMIA

Key Concept:

Hypoxia is a very dangerous situation and, if not quickly corrected, can lead to permanent injury or death.

As you learned in Chapter 1, hypoxemia means that there is a low level of oxygen in the blood. Hypoxemia is a leading cause of hypoxia—not enough oxygen in the cells to keep metabolism working properly.

Hypoxia can be caused by a number of problems, including:

■ Not enough oxygen reaching the alveoli. This can be the result of suffocation, shallow breathing, or being at high altitude.

■ Decreased diffusion of oxygen through the alveoli. This can be the result of pulmonary fibrosis or pulmonary (alveolar) edema.

■ Shunt or increased blood flow compared to ventilation. This can be the result of pneumonia.

■ Anemia. This can be the result of bleeding or a disease of the blood (erythrocytes).

■ Carbon monoxide poisoning. This can be the result of inhaling carbon monoxide produced by a house fire or from automobile exhaust.

■ Heart failure so that not enough blood reaches the tissues. This can be the result of heart disease or a heart attack.

■ Cyanide poisoning, which prevents the cells from using oxygen. Cyanide poisoning most commonly happens when smoke from a house fire is inhaled.

Regardless of the cause(s) of hypoxemia, it must be rapidly corrected. Most of the following discussion in this chapter deals with tests to determine lung or heart disease or treatments to correct hypoxemia.

■ CARDIOPULMONARY TESTS

Cardiopulmonary tests are tests of the airways, lungs, heart, and/or blood. They are often needed to diagnose a patient's disease. Additionally, they are used to evaluate how the patient is responding to the care he or she is receiving. Based on the results of the cardiopulmonary tests, the physician may decide to increase the number of treatments, change them, or discontinue them.

Pulse Oximetry

The pulse oximetry (SpO_2) test is used to determine if a patient is hypoxic. The procedure is easy to perform and is widely used to measure the saturation of the erythrocytes' (RBCs) hemoglobin with oxygen. The measurement is given as a percentage (%). The saturation percentage represents how full the arterial blood is with oxygen. A pulse oximetry value of 95% or more is expected in a normal person. In most patients with cardiopulmonary disease, it is desirable to have a pulse oximetry value of at least 90%. This means that the RBCs are at least 90% full of oxygen. The physician usually writes an order to keep the patient's pulse oximeter value at a certain safe level (for example, 92%).

The pulse oximeter is able to measure the hemoglobin saturation through the patient's skin, so there is no need to take a blood sample. Many pulse oximeter units also give a reading for the patient's heart rate. A pulse oximeter device includes the measuring instrument and the patient attachment sensor (Figure 3-1). Often the sensor is attached to a patient's finger tip. Different sensors attach to the ear, toe, heel, or bridge of nose. The patient may have a single measurement taken, or may have the unit left on for a prolonged time to monitor reaction to treatment. Commonly the pulse oximeter value is checked when supplemental oxygen is started or changed. If a pulse oximeter is used for patient monitoring, it usually has a visual and audible alarm system. You need to understand how the alarm works.

Current models of pulse oximeters will give inaccurate values if used on patients with carbon monoxide poisoning. The devices should not be used with

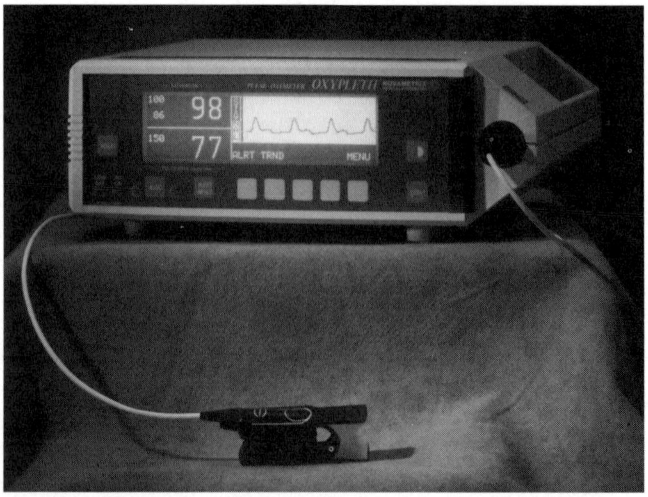

■■ **Key Concept:** *Notify the RCP or RN if the patient's pulse oximetry value is less than what the physician orders.* ■■

■■ **Key Concept:** *If the pulse oximeter alarm goes off (with a sound and/or light signal), you must check the patient and get help if needed.* ■■

Figure 3-1 A typical pulse oximeter with a finger sensor. (Courtesy of Novametrix Medical Systems, Inc., Wallingford, CT)

these patients. Additionally, pulse oximetry values may not be accurate in these situations:

1. The patient has poor blood flow to the sensor site or low blood pressure.
2. The patient is wearing nail polish when a finger sensor is used.
3. There are bright lights shining on the sensor.
4. The patient has dark skin color.

Get the RCP or RN whenever you have difficulty in using a pulse oximeter.

Arterial Blood Gases

The arterial blood gases (ABGs) test is used to evaluate a patient's arterial blood oxygen level (PaO_2). Additionally, it is used to measure how much carbon dioxide is in the patient's arterial blood ($PaCO_2$), his or her pH (acid-base level), and several related values. The arterial blood gas test and its results are better than pulse oximetry in many patient situations. This is because it better evaluates the patient's breathing and heart function by measuring both the oxygen level and the carbon dioxide level.

An arterial blood gas test involves taking a sample of blood from one of the patient's arteries (Figure 1-18). Only a properly trained RCP, RN, physician, or **medical laboratory technician** can draw such a blood sample. You may need to assist in the procedure by:

1. Making sure the patient has been wearing his or her oxygen system for at least 15 minutes.
2. Holding the puncture site for at least 5 minutes to prevent bleeding.
3. Getting a plastic bag or cup with ice and water if the sample must be taken to the laboratory.
4. Promptly taking the blood sample, in ice water, to the laboratory for analysis. (In some cases, the blood sample is analyzed at the patient's bedside with a portable blood gas analyzer.)

■ *medical laboratory technician: a person who, under the supervision of a medical technologist or physician, performs various tests on human blood, tissue, and fluids for diagnostic and research purposes*

Chest X-Ray

Most patients with heart or lung problems will have an x-ray taken of the chest, neck, or abdomen. The x-ray procedure sends energy waves through the body to a large piece of special photographic film. The internal organs such as the heart and lungs can be seen in the shape of shadows on the film. It is recommended that a chest x-ray film be seen, if possible. The **radiologic technologist** (also called x-ray technician) positions the patient and runs the equipment to perform the procedure. You may be needed to help transport the patient to the Radiology Department or help position the patient if the x-ray procedure is done with the patient in his or her bed.

■ *radiologic technologist: a person who, under the supervision of a physician or radiologist, operates radiologic (x-ray) equipment*

Electrocardiogram

An electrocardiogram (ECG or EKG) is done to determine the patient's heart rate and rhythm. Certain heart conditions can be diagnosed by ECG results. A 12-lead ECG is done for diagnostic purposes. It requires that a series of electrodes be placed properly on the patient's chest, arms, and legs (Figure 3-2). In some cases the patient must be continuously monitored for heart function. This involves the use of three chest electrodes.

In many hospitals, an ECG technician or RCP will perform all electrocardiograms. However, your institution may choose to train you to perform them. If the patient is having heart function continuously monitored on your patient care unit, the ECG monitor will have a visual and audible alarm. It is important that you understand the alarm system.

■ **Key Concept:** *If the ECG alarm goes off, you must check the patient and get help if needed.* ■

Pulmonary Function Testing (PFT)

Airway and lung function are determined through a series of specific tests performed by RCPs. The results of these tests help the physician determine the patient's diagnosis and response to care. Some tests can be performed at the

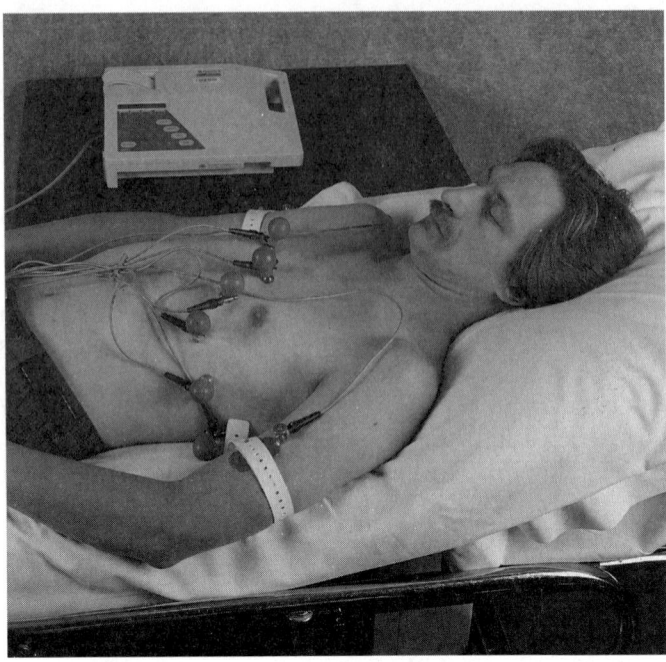

Figure 3-2 Proper placement of the six precordial leads to obtain an electrocardiogram tracing. Placement of the two arm leads can also be seen. Unseen are the leg leads attached to the lower legs.

patient's bedside with portable instruments. These tests commonly measure how fast a patient can exhale, tidal volume, the maximum volume that can be exhaled, and the strength of the inspiratory and expiratory muscles. Other tests require that the patient be transported to the pulmonary function laboratory.

Sputum Sample

Most patients with bronchitis and pneumonia produce large amounts of mucus (pulmonary secretions). Mucus can plug the airways, so it is very important that these secretions be removed. The mucus contains the organism infecting the patient. When mucus is coughed out, it is called *sputum.* The physician usually orders that a sputum sample be obtained in order to determine what organism(s) is causing the patient's infection. A sputum sample may also be obtained to look for cancer cells from the lungs. Most of the time an RCP or RN is called upon to get the sputum sample. You may be asked to get a particular type of sterile container for the patient to cough into. You may also be asked, as the PCT, to collect the sputum sample by encouraging the patient to cough into the container at the bedside. (The cough and deep breathing procedure is included later in this chapter. Laboratory and clinical checkoff lists on the procedure are included in the Appendix.)

■■■■ OXYGEN THERAPY

Oxygen therapy involves the patient being given a prescribed amount of oxygen greater than the 21% found in room air. The physician will order that a patient receive supplemental oxygen when the patient's oxygen level is low. Examples of conditions causing hypoxemia include, but are not limited to, shortness of breath, heart disease, chronic obstructive lung disease, and pneumonia. By law, supplemental oxygen is a drug. The patient's physician must write an order for how much oxygen is to be given to the patient and what type of oxygen mask or other device should be used to give the oxygen. The physician may also write an order for the RCP to evaluate the patient and determine the correct oxygen percent and system. Many types of masks and other devices are used to give the patient supplemental oxygen; some of the more common types are described in this section. Usually the RCP sets up the oxygen delivery system, makes sure that it is working, and evaluates the patient's response. However, there are times

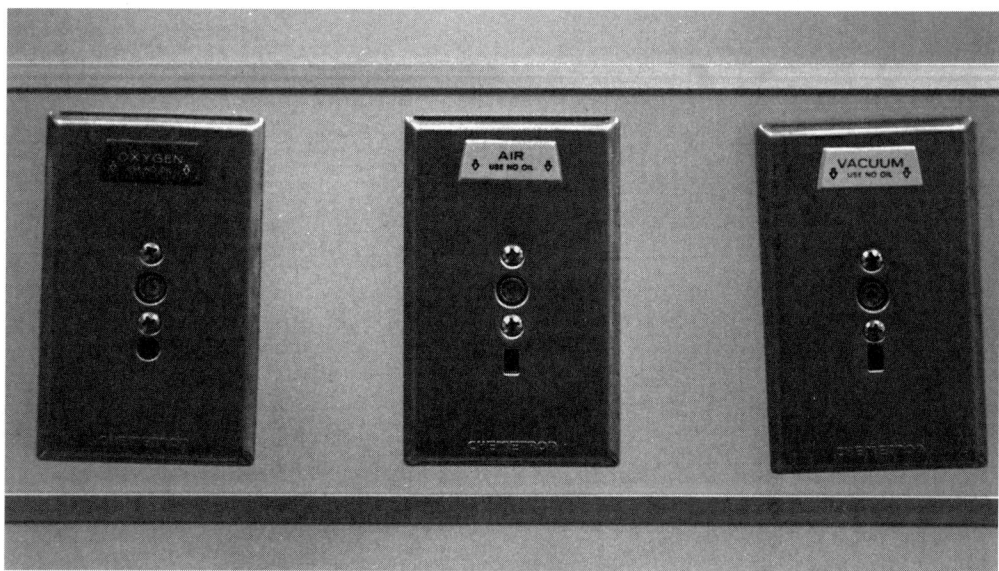

Figure 3-3   A bank of three quick-connect fittings, as seen in many patient care rooms. An oxygen flowmeter would connect to the left outlet, an air flowmeter would connect in the center outlet, and a vacuum system would connect in the right fitting.

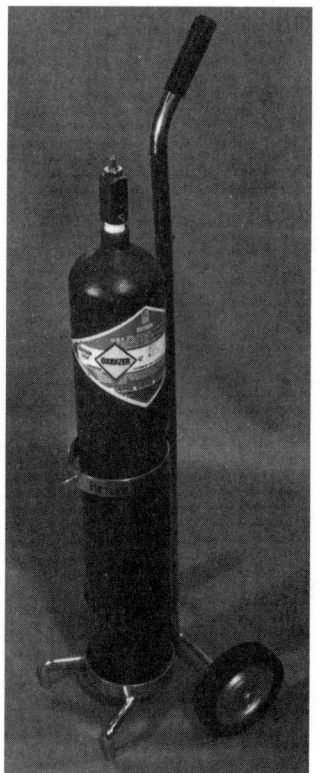

Figure 3-4   An "E" size tank of oxygen in its cart. The top part of the tank is called the *stem*. A regulator is attached to it to measure the pressure within the tank and allow the oxygen to flow out in a controlled manner.

when a trained RN or paramedic will set up the system. The RCP may then be called to ensure that it is functioning properly. You may be trained by your employer to maintain the proper functioning of the oxygen system. Your employer may expect that you can assist with some oxygen administration procedures. (Laboratory and clinical checkoff lists for several oxygen administration device procedures are included in the Appendix.)

Wall Oxygen Outlets

Oxygen is piped throughout most hospitals and extended care facilities by piping within the walls. The patient outlets for oxygen are made by several manufacturers. Only oxygen flowmeters made by the same manufacturer will fit into them. Practice is required to connect a flowmeter into the outlet and remove it properly. Make sure that you read the label on the outlet. Many rooms have banks of outlets for one or more oxygen sources, piped-in compressed air, and one or more vacuum ports for suctioning (Figure 3-3). Be sure to connect into the proper outlet.

Portable Oxygen Tanks

Small tanks of oxygen are available in most nursing units or through the Respiratory Care Department to transport a patient who needs continuous oxygen. The contents of the tank are confirmed by the word OXYGEN printed on the tank label. Additionally, oxygen tanks are painted green in the United States. The tanks are typically a size labeled as "E" (Figure 3-4). The full oxygen tank is pressurized to at least 2,000 psi (pounds per square inch of tank surface). Figure 3-5 shows one type of regulator used with oxygen tanks to reduce the pressure and allow a controlled flow of oxygen. A tank is considered empty and should be replaced when its pressure is less than 500 psi. (This "empty" tank is still highly pressurized and contains quite a lot of oxygen.)

For safety, it is important to keep the tank from being knocked over. It must be kept in a tank cart, chained to the wall, or in a tank holder on a wheelchair or gurney. An oxygen tank should not be placed near open flame or anything flammable, such as gasoline or petroleum products.

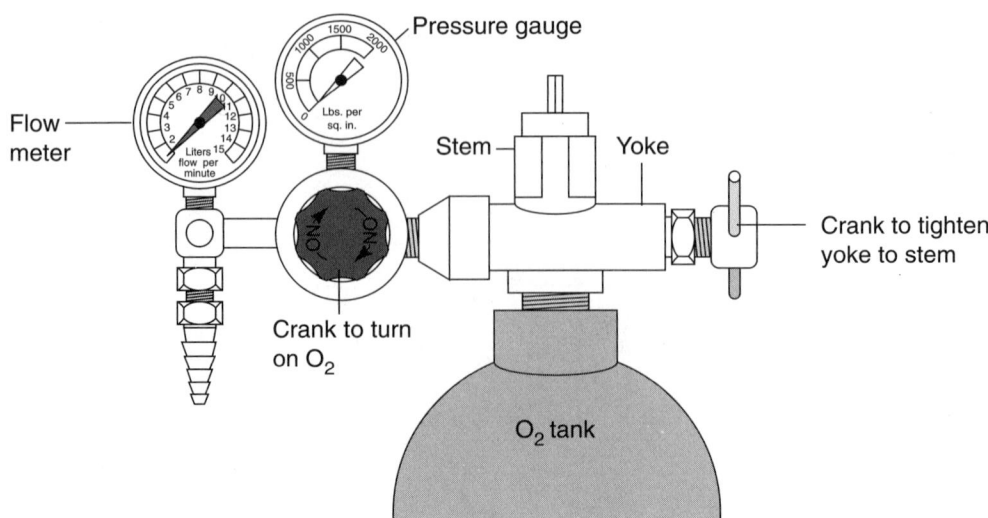

Figure 3-5   One type of regulator for an "E" size oxygen tank. The gauge on the right shows the pressure within the tank. The gauge on the left shows the oxygen flow in liters per minute (LPM). A knob is rotated clockwise to turn on the gas flow. Oxygen exits from the threaded opening beneath the left gauge. An oxygen nipple adapter has been added so that small-bore tubing can be attached. Other equipment can be screwed onto the oxygen outlet as needed. Turning the knob counterclockwise turns off the gas flow. The right part of the regulator, called the *yoke,* attaches it to the stem of the tank. The handle on the far right is used to tighten or loosen the regulator from the tank. A tank wrench is connected to the valve stem.

Procedures are provided later in this chapter for preparing a new oxygen tank or preparing an oxygen tank for patient transport. Laboratory and clinical checkoff lists on these procedures are included in the Appendix.

Patient Safety When Oxygen Is in Use

Oxygen supports burning. Additionally, the oxygen in wall piping or portable tanks is under great pressure. Any leak will cause a great deal of oxygen to come out rapidly. An open flame or spark can start a fire that will rapidly burn because of the extra oxygen in the area.

The following safety rules apply when oxygen is in use:

■ An "OXYGEN IN USE" sign must be posted in the room of any patient using oxygen. The sign should also warn against using open flames, electrical appliances, or smoking.

■ Patients and family members must be warned that oxygen is being used and told of the preceding prohibitions.

■ Do not attempt to force any flowmeter, regulator, or other device into any oxygen source. This could jam the oxygen source open and cause high-pressure oxygen to leak out.

■ Oxygen tanks must be stored securely so that they will not fall over.

■ *Always* check the contents of any tank of gas. The label will state its contents. Also check the color of the tank. Oxygen tanks are painted green in the United States.

■ Get the RCP if any oxygen equipment or other respiratory care equipment is not working properly or is making any unusual sounds. Many respiratory care devices have built-in audible and visual alarms if there is a problem.

In case of fire in an area where oxygen is in use, get the patients to safety as soon as possible. Call a fire emergency. The piped oxygen in the wall can be turned off at one of the zone valves. Have your instructor or supervisor show you where the zone valve is and how to shut off the oxygen to your nursing unit if there is a fire.

■■ **Key Concept:** *If there should be a fire in a room when oxygen is in use, it is critical to get the patient out of the room as soon as safely possible.* ■■

■■ **Key Concept:** *Supplemental oxygen, by any system, must be kept on the patient at all times. Removing it can result in a dangerous drop in the patient's oxygen level.* ■■

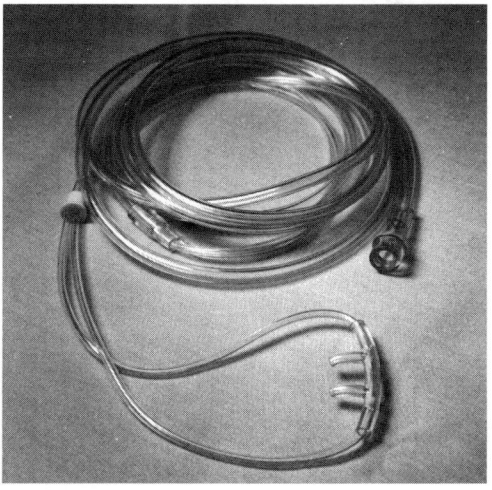

Figure 3-6 A typical adult-size nasal cannula

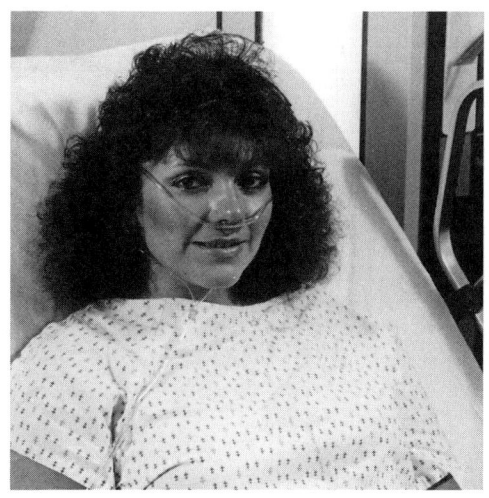

Figure 3-7 A nasal cannula placed properly on a patient

Nasal Cannula

A nasal cannula oxygen delivery system is a small-diameter (bore) plastic hose (tube) that ends in two prongs that fit into the nostrils (Figures 3-6 and 3-7). Cannulas come in adult and pediatric sizes. The non-patient end of the cannula connects to an adapter on the oxygen flowmeter or to a humidifier on the flowmeter. The physician must order how many liters per minute of oxygen are to go to the patient. Make sure the ordered flow of oxygen is going to the patient. Most patients find a nasal cannula to be comfortable. However, sometimes the plastic tubing rubs on the skin of the nostrils or over the ears. Patients can eat and drink with the cannula on. A nasal cannula is used primarily to give low to moderate amounts of oxygen to patients with a stable breathing pattern. A patient with blocked nasal passages or unstable breathing should not use a nasal cannula. Contact the RCP or RN about the situation.

Simple Oxygen Mask

A simple, basic oxygen mask fits over the patient's nose and mouth and extends to the chin. It has a small-diameter tube that connects to the adapter on a flowmeter or a humidifier on a flowmeter. Masks come in different sizes for adults and children. A stretchable strap holds the mask on the patient's head (Figures 3-8 and 3-9). The physician must order how many liters per minute of oxygen are to go to the patient. Make sure the ordered flow of oxygen is going to the patient. A simple oxygen mask will deliver moderate amounts of oxygen because the mask acts as a reservoir. It is preferred for patients who need more oxygen or who have an unstable breathing pattern.

To eat or drink, the patient will have to briefly lift this or any oxygen mask with each bite. Alternatively, the physician may order that a nasal cannula be used during meals.

Key Concept:
Patients should never go without their supplemental oxygen during meals or on any other occasion.

Air Entrainment Mask

The air entrainment mask is also known as a *venturi mask, venti mask,* and *high airflow with oxygen enrichment (HAFOE) mask.* This mask comes in adult and child sizes and is modified from a simple mask. A small-diameter oxygen hose is connected to a flowmeter or humidifier on a flowmeter, as with the simple mask (Figures 3-10 and 3-11). However, this mask is special in that different, specific percentages of oxygen can be delivered through it. A larger plastic tube hangs down from the mask. It acts as a blender to mix entrained (pulled-in) room air with supplemental oxygen to get the ordered oxygen percentage. Several

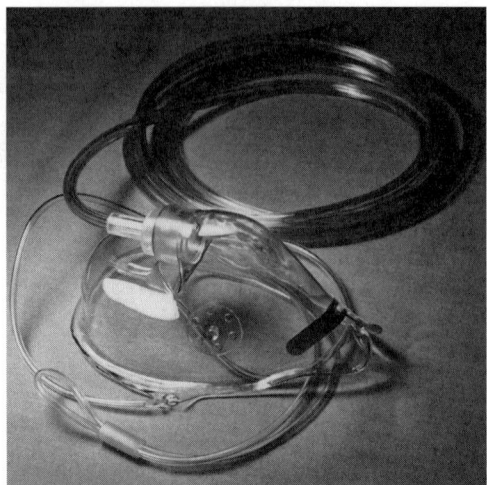

Figure 3-8   A typical adult-size simple oxygen mask

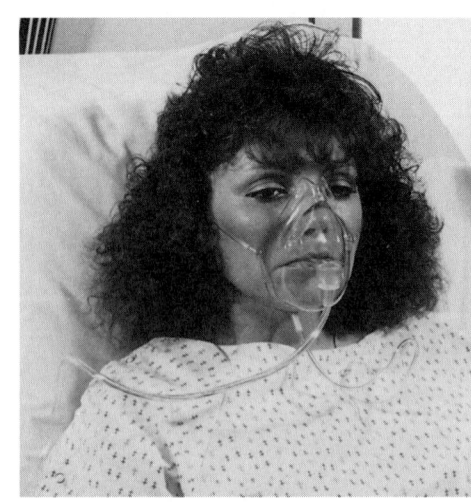

Figure 3-9   A simple oxygen mask placed correctly on a patient

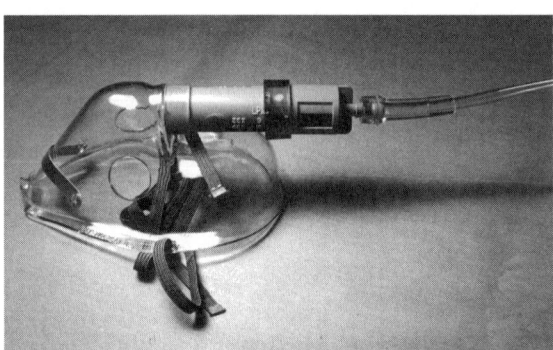

Figure 3-10   A typical air entrainment mask

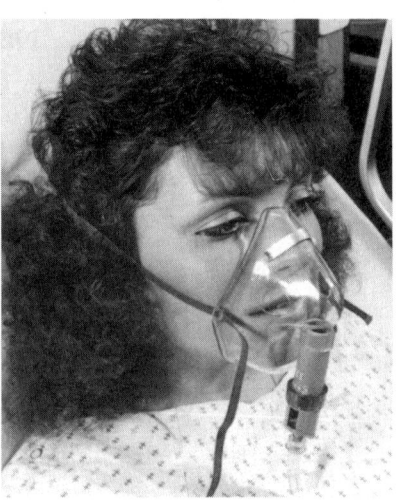

Figure 3-11   An air entrainment mask properly placed on a patient. Make sure that the bottom tube is not covered by bedding.

different oxygen percentages, ranking from low to moderate, can be set on the mask. The physician should order what oxygen percentage is needed. Only the RCP should set this mask up on the patient and make sure that it is operating properly. PCT responsibilities may include:

1. Making sure that the patient does not play with or move the mask, as he or she may accidentally change the oxygen percentage.
2. Making sure that the patient does not cover the mask with bedding, as this will change the oxygen percentage.

Nonrebreather Mask

A nonrebreather mask is modified from a simple mask. It also has a small-diameter tube to connect to the oxygen flowmeter (Figures 3-12 and 3-13). The mask has one or two plastic flaps on the sides that let the patient breathe out but do not allow room air to be brought in. Below the mask hangs a reservoir bag for oxygen. The reservoir bag and special mask ensure that a high percent-

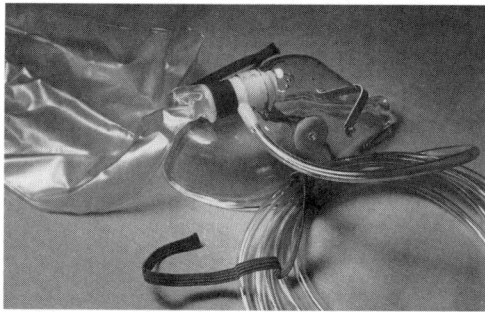

Figure 3-12 A typical nonrebreathing mask. Note the round flaps that prevent room air from being inhaled.

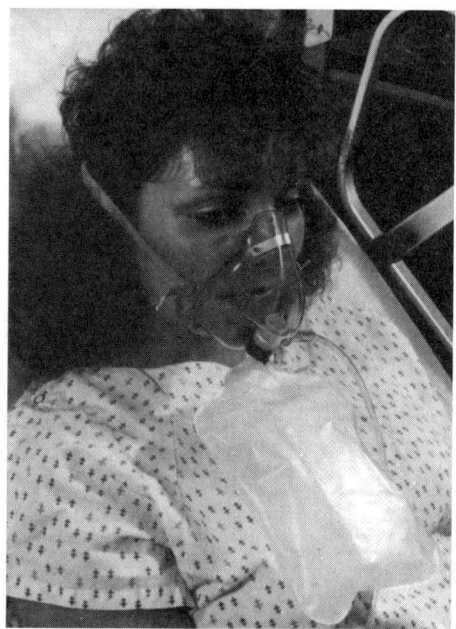

Figure 3-13 A nonrebreathing mask placed correctly on a patient. Make sure that the reservoir bag does not collapse more than half on inspiration. The bag should not be covered by bedding.

age of oxygen is delivered to the patient. Only the most hypoxic patients should be using this type of oxygen mask. The RCP should be the only person to set this mask up on the patient and make sure that it is operating correctly. You must make sure that the patient does not cover the reservoir bag with bedding. The reservoir bag must not collapse. Call the RCP if the reservoir bag does not stay at least half full when the patient breathes in.

Aerosol Mask

An aerosol mask has two modifications from a simple mask (Figure 3-14). First, a large opening is cut into each side of the mask for the patient to exhale through. Second, and most important, a large-diameter (bore) adapter is on the bottom of the mask, so that large-diameter tubing can be added. This tubing goes to a device that generates an **aerosol** of water. The aerosol is usually carried to the patient by supplemental oxygen. You must make sure that the patient wears the mask and that aerosol can be seen to come out of the ports on the mask at all times. Call the RCP if no aerosol is coming out of the mask.

■ **aerosol:** *microscopic particles of water or medicine suspended in a gas or air; also called a* mist *or* spray

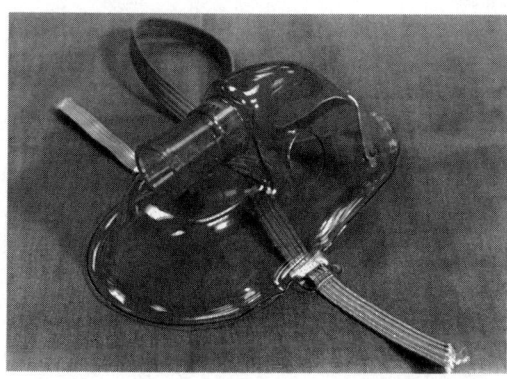

Figure 3-14 A typical adult-size aerosol mask

Tracheostomy Mask

A special tracheostomy mask is used to give supplemental oxygen and aerosol to a patient who has a tracheostomy (Figure 3-15). The mask part covers the patient's tracheostomy tube so that aerosol and oxygen are inhaled. The large-diameter adapter on the mask connects to large-diameter tubing that goes to an aerosol generator. Oxygen or compressed air pushes the aerosol to the mask. You must make sure that the mask stays in place by being strapped around the patient's neck. Call the RCP if no aerosol is seen coming out of the mask.

▬▬▬ HUMIDITY AND AEROSOL THERAPY

Normally, the upper airway adds water vapor to inhaled air. However, many patients are not able to humidify the air properly. Because of this, moisture is added by a respiratory care device to the patient's inhaled air or oxygen.

Humidifying the Airway

■ *humidity: dampness; the amount of moisture in the atmosphere or a room*

■ *humidifier: a device that keeps the atmosphere moist by converting liquid water to water vapor*

Pure oxygen coming from a wall outlet or a tank is dry. Patients with normal upper airways can tolerate small amounts of dry oxygen without any problem. However, **humidity** is usually added for comfort. The RCP will usually install a **humidifier** in the oxygen delivery system. The type shown in Figure 3-16 is designed to connect to the small-diameter tubing used with a nasal cannula or simple oxygen mask. When operating normally, the oxygen will bubble through the water in the reservoir and go out the tubing to the patient. If the tubing is kinked, the oxygen will not exit. Pressure will build up in the unit and vent out of a pressure relief valve. This will cause a whistling or popping sound. PCT actions are to:

1. Make sure that sterile water is within the reservoir jar.
2. Listen for an abnormal whistling sound. Call the RCP if the humidifier is whistling or popping or the water level is low.

■ *nebulizer: a medical device that uses compressed air or oxygen to convert liquid water to an aerosol*

Another type of humidifier, shown in Figure 3-17, is called a **nebulizer** and makes an aerosol of very small water droplets. Either piped-in oxygen or compressed air powers the unit. It is designed to connect to large-diameter tubing like that used with an aerosol mask or tracheostomy mask. As with humidifiers,

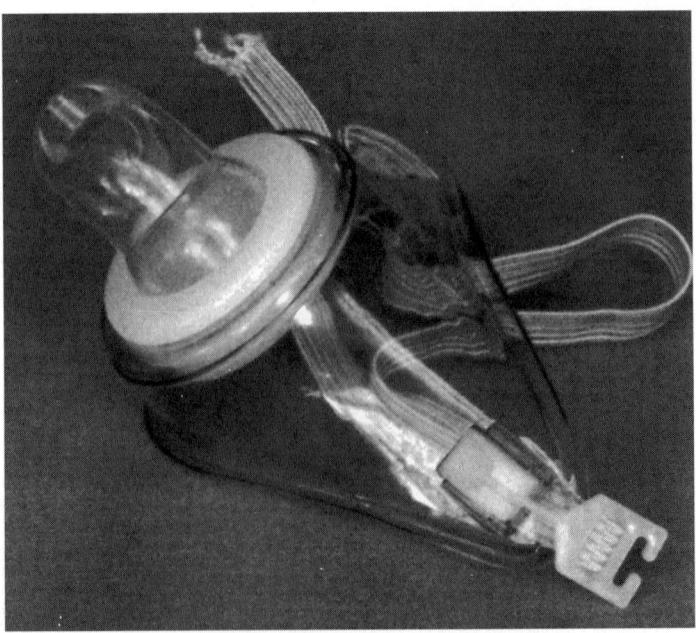

Figure 3-15 A typical adult-size tracheostomy (aerosol) mask

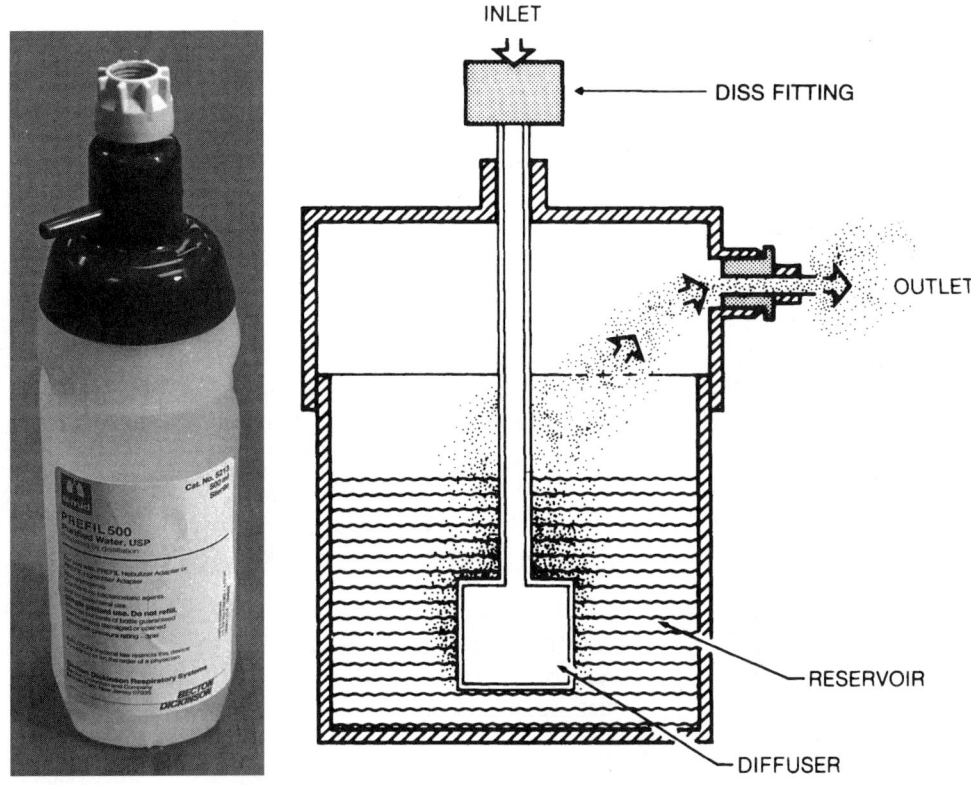

Figure 3-16 A photograph and functional diagram of a water-filled, bubble-type humidifier

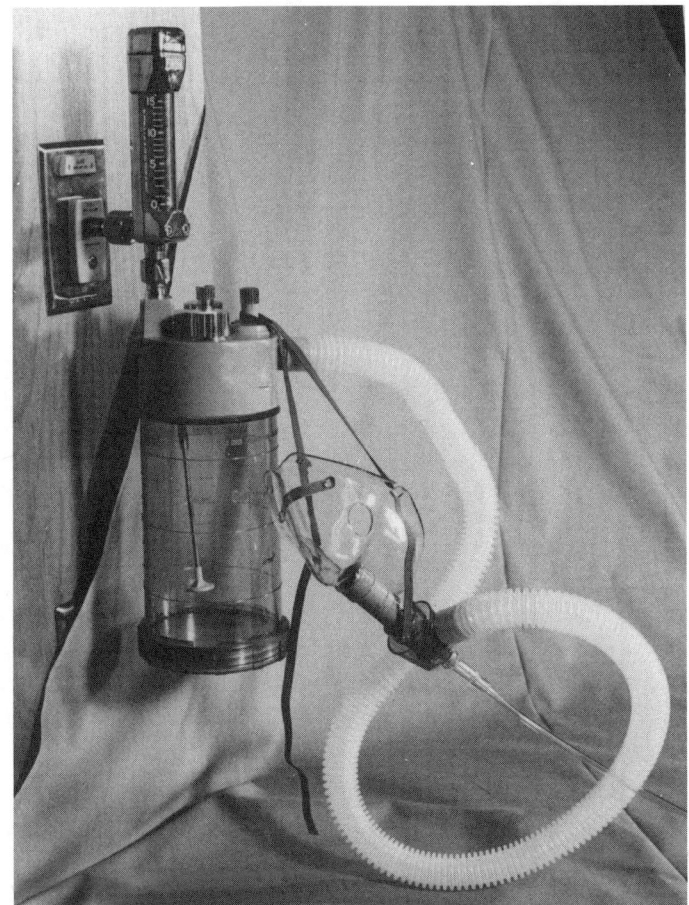

Figure 3-17 A water-filled, large-volume nebulizer. The attached large-bore tubing carries the aerosol to the venturi mask.

water must be in the reservoir jar and the gas must exit properly or the pressure will cause a whistling sound as it leaks out. PCT actions are to:

1. Make sure that sterile water is within the reservoir jar.
2. Listen for an abnormal whistling or popping sound.
3. Check that an aerosol is going to the patient's face mask. Call the RCP if the nebulizer is making an unusual sound or the water level is low.

Aerosolized Medications

Many patients with lung disease inhale medications into their airways and lungs. There are a number of different types of medications designed to relax the tight airways of asthmatics, liquefy secretions, fight infection, numb the airways, or treat airway edema. The RCP usually delivers these medications through a **metered dose inhaler (MDI)** or small-volume nebulizer (Figures 3-18 and 3-19). Sometimes the RN gives the medication and sometimes the patient may be allowed to take a medication by himself or herself. Because of state laws regulating who can administer medications, you cannot.

ARTIFICIAL AIRWAYS

If a patient with any kind of artificial airway has it come out, or has difficulty breathing, get the RCP or RN immediately. Artificial airways include the oropharyngeal airway, the nasopharyngeal airway, the endotracheal tube, and the tracheostomy tube.

Oropharyngeal Airway

An oropharyngeal airway is a firm, plastic device placed into the mouth of a patient who is unconscious. It holds the tongue forward so that it does not block the back of the throat. Some airways are hollow; others have deep grooves for breathing through. Examples are shown in Figure 3-20. Airway placement in a patient is shown in Figure 3-21. The oropharyngeal airway is usually placed into the patient by an RCP or RN. When the correct size airway is properly placed into the unconscious patient, his or her breathing should be easier. PCT actions may include:

1. Obtaining the type of airway requested by the RCP or RN.
2. Making sure that the patient is breathing satisfactorily with it in place.

Key Concept:
Report any patient's complaint of a medication reaction to the RN or RCP.

■ *metered dose inhaler (MDI): a medical device that uses pressurized gas in a canister to convert a liquid medication to an aerosolized medication for inhalation*

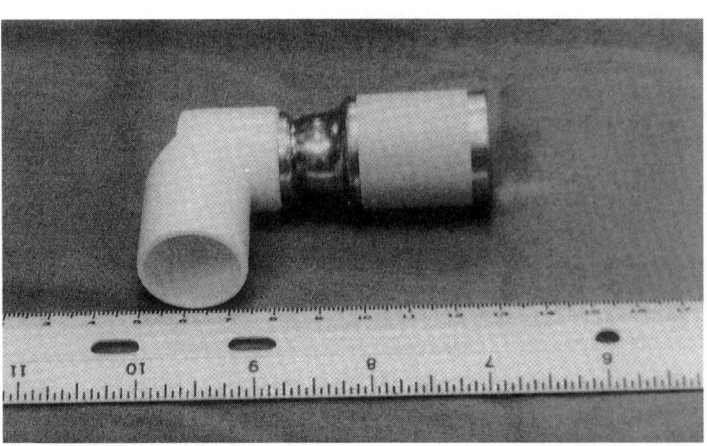 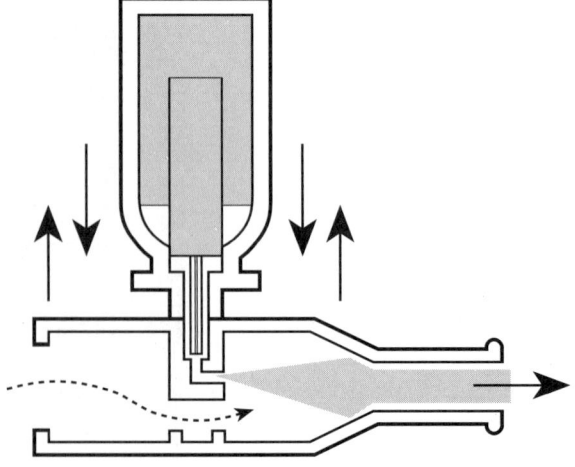

Figure 3-18   A photograph and functional diagram of a metered dose inhaler. Liquid medication and compressed gas are contained within the canister.

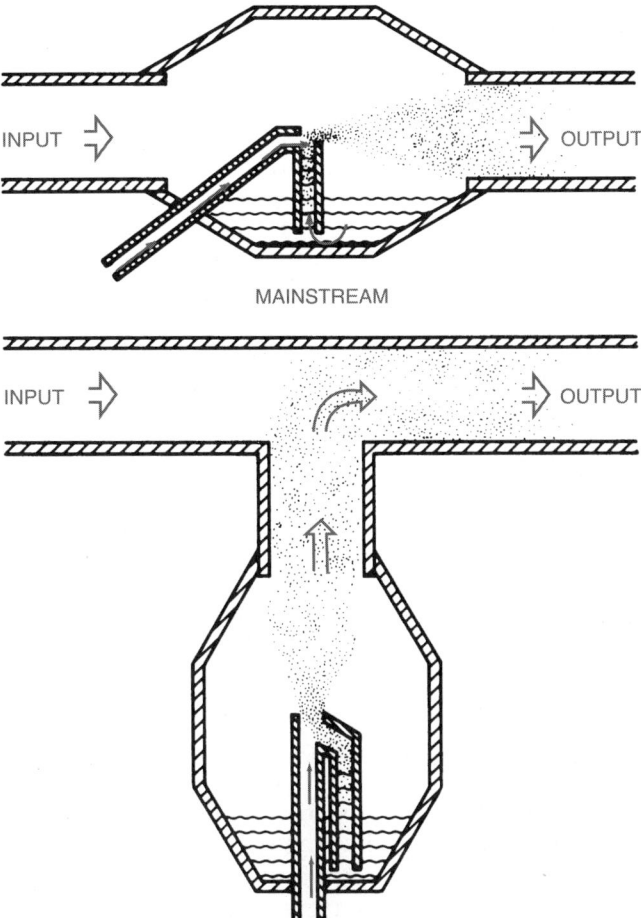

Figure 3-19 Functional diagrams of a mainstream and a sidestream medication nebulizer. Compressed oxygen or air from the wall outlet converts the liquid medication into an aerosol.

MAINSTREAM

SIDESTREAM

INPUT OUTPUT

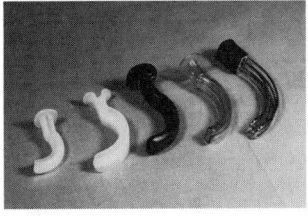

Figure 3-20 Several types and sizes of oropharyngeal airways

If the airway comes out, or if the patient should have any gagging or difficulty breathing, report it immediately to the RCP or RN.

Nasopharyngeal Airway

A soft, hollow, rubber nasopharyngeal airway is placed into the nasal passage of a patient who may be either conscious or unconscious. This airway is shown in Figure 3-22 and its placement into a patient is shown in Figure 3-23. The nasopharyngeal airway has two purposes. First, it extends to the oropharynx and pushes the tongue forward to keep the airway open. Second, it provides a route for placing a suction catheter to remove secretions from the throat or the trachea. The nasopharyngeal airway is usually well tolerated and should not cause any gagging in an awake patient. The airway is usually inserted by an RCP or RN. PCT actions may include:

1. Obtaining the size airway requested by the RCP or RN.

2. Making sure that the patient is breathing satisfactorily with it in place.

If the airway comes out, or if the patient should have any gagging or difficulty breathing, report it immediately to the RCP or RN.

Endotracheal Tube

A flexible, hollow, plastic endotracheal tube is placed into the patient's trachea to provide a secure airway. With this tube in place, the patient can breathe spontaneously, or mechanical ventilation can be applied. Additionally, a suction

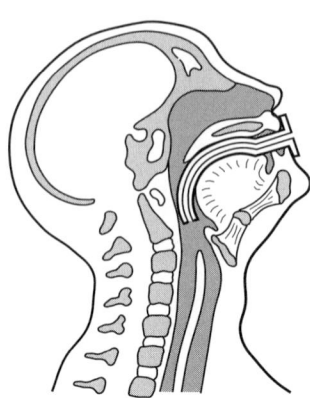

Figure 3-21 A cutaway drawing of the head showing the proper placement of an oropharyngeal airway behind the tongue. The patient can still breathe around the artificial airway.

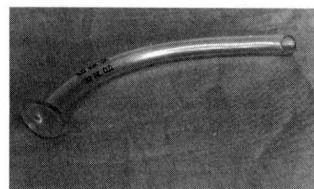

Figure 3-22 A nasopharyngeal airway

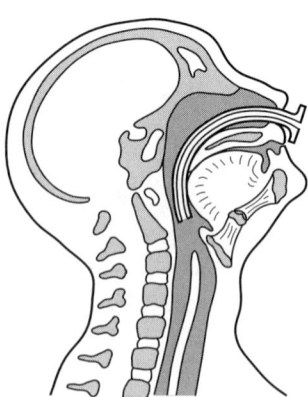

Figure 3-23 A cutaway drawing of the head showing the proper placement of a nasopharyngeal airway behind the tongue. The patient can still breathe around the artificial airway.

catheter can be placed through it to remove airway secretions. The patient end of the tube has a balloon around it called a *cuff*. The cuff is inflated or deflated with a syringe through a small attached tube. The outside end of the tube has an adapter that fits to a resuscitation bag or mechanical ventilator. See Figure 3-24 for the tube and Figure 3-25 for its placement into a patient. Very sick patients with serious cardiopulmonary problems will have an endotracheal tube placed into them. Often the patient is moved to the intensive care unit for close monitoring. The endotracheal tube is usually placed into the patient by a physician or specially trained RCP. The procedure is called *intubation* and is often done in an emergency situation, such as during a cardiopulmonary resuscitation effort. PCT actions may include:

1. Assisting with ventilating the patient.
2. Obtaining the correct size endotracheal tube.

If the tube is partially or completely pulled out, or if the patient is having difficulty breathing, call the RCP or RN immediately. Do not attempt to put the endotracheal tube back in.

Tracheostomy Tube

A tracheostomy tube is a shorter version of the endotracheal tube. It is placed into the patient's trachea by a surgeon through an opening cut into the base of the neck in front. The tracheostomy tube is usually placed into a patient who needs a permanent artificial airway. With this tube in place, the patient can breathe spontaneously, or mechanical ventilation can be applied. Additionally, a suction catheter can be placed through it to remove airway secretions. Conscious patients find a tracheostomy tube more comfortable than an endotracheal tube. Additionally, the patient with a tracheostomy tube can eat and drink. The patient end of the tube has a balloon around it called a *cuff*. The cuff is inflated or deflated with a syringe through a small attached tube. The outside end of the tube has an adapter that fits to a resuscitation bag or mechanical ventilator. Tracheostomy tubes may be made of a firm plastic or metal. Some are only a single tube; others have an outer tube and a removable inner tube or cannula (Figure 3-26). Depending on where you work and your job description, you may be expected to assist in care of the tracheostomy site or routine replacement of the tracheostomy tube. This care may include the following:

1. Gathering the needed equipment and supplies: new tracheostomy tube, sterile 4″ × 4″ gauze pads, sterile scissors, sterile gloves, 10-mL syringe, sterile water-soluble lubricant, antibiotic ointment, sterile basin with sterile water.
2. Removing and replacing the tracheostomy mask.
3. Monitoring the patient's pulse oximetry value and vital signs.

You should make sure that a replacement tracheostomy tube of the same size is kept in the patient's room if needed. If the tube should come out, or if the patient has difficulty breathing, get the RCP or RN immediately. Do not attempt to put the tracheostomy tube back into the patient.

Securing the Artificial Airway

All of the airways described here must be secured to keep them from being coughed or pulled out by the patient. Usually a strap made of adhesive tape or special string ties is used to secure the airway in the correct position. An oropharyngeal airway is usually held in place with adhesive tape to both cheeks. A nasopharyngeal airway is usually held in place with tape across the bridge of the nose. An endotracheal tube is commonly held in place with adhesive tape around it and to the upper lip. Cloth straps may also be used to keep it from sliding in or out. Cloth straps that tie behind the patient's neck are used to secure a tracheostomy tube. The RCP or RN will secure the airway in its proper place. You may need to assist by getting tape or ties.

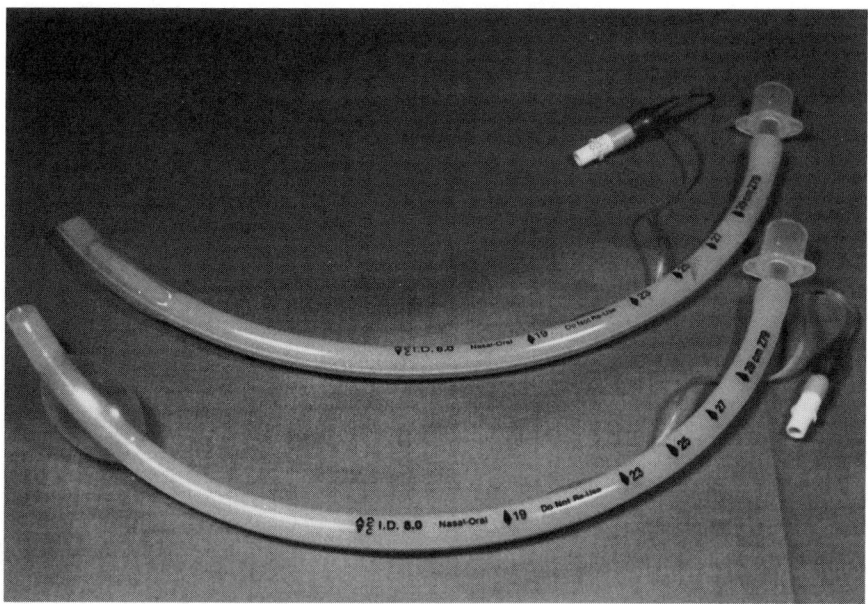

Figure 3-24 Two adult-size endotracheal tubes. The cuff on the bottom one has been inflated through the attached small-diameter tube.

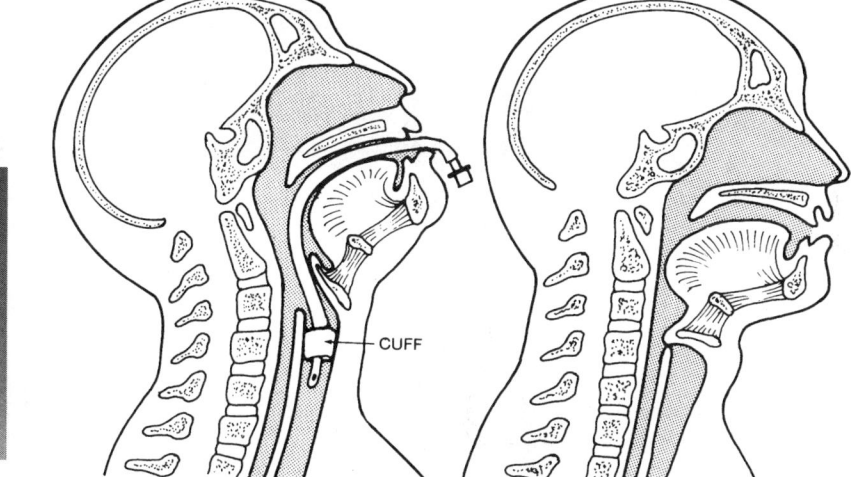

Figure 3-25 A cutaway drawing of the head showing the proper placement of an endotracheal tube through the mouth and into the trachea. The cuff is inflated to seal the airway. The patient will breathe through the tube.

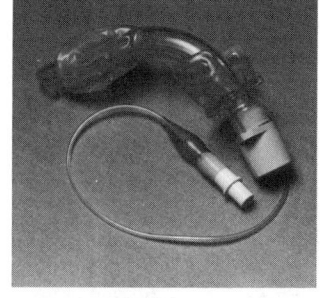

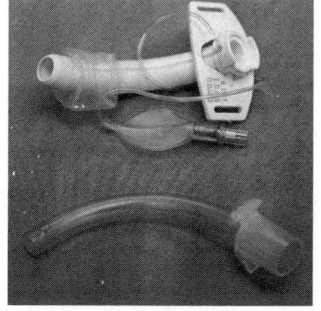

Figure 3-26 Two typical adult-size plastic tracheostomy tubes with deflated cuffs. The right one has a removable inner cannula.

Mouth Care

Care must be taken when performing mouth care on a patient with any type of artificial airway. The tube must not be moved deeper into the patient or pulled out from its proper position. Oropharyngeal (mouth) suctioning can usually be done along either or both cheeks. This procedure is discussed later.

■■■■ CARDIOPULMONARY RESUSCITATION

It is very likely that you will witness attempts at cardiopulmonary resuscitation (CPR) while at work. You may be called upon to participate in it. Most employers require that employees who work in patient care areas learn basic CPR. If not,

■■■ **Key Concept:** *Know the steps in performing CPR and how to call the CPR team.* ■■

it is highly recommended that you take it upon yourself to learn CPR. You may save the life of a patient, friend, or family member.

Basic CPR teaches you to do mouth-to-mouth ventilation if a patient is not breathing. However, an artificial ventilation device is preferred because supplemental oxygen can be added to it to correct hypoxemia. Your employer may expect that you can assist with a CPR attempt by using either a mouth-to-valve mask (pocket mask) or resuscitation bag and CPR mask to ventilate a patient. Figures 3-27 and 3-28 show the mouth-to-valve unit. It is made up of a patient face mask, gas flow valve, and mouthpiece for you to blow through. Figures 3-29 and 3-30 show the resuscitation bag and mask. The bags and face masks come in different sizes based on the size of the patient. The bag also has a gas flow valve and small-diameter hose through which oxygen can be added. Both

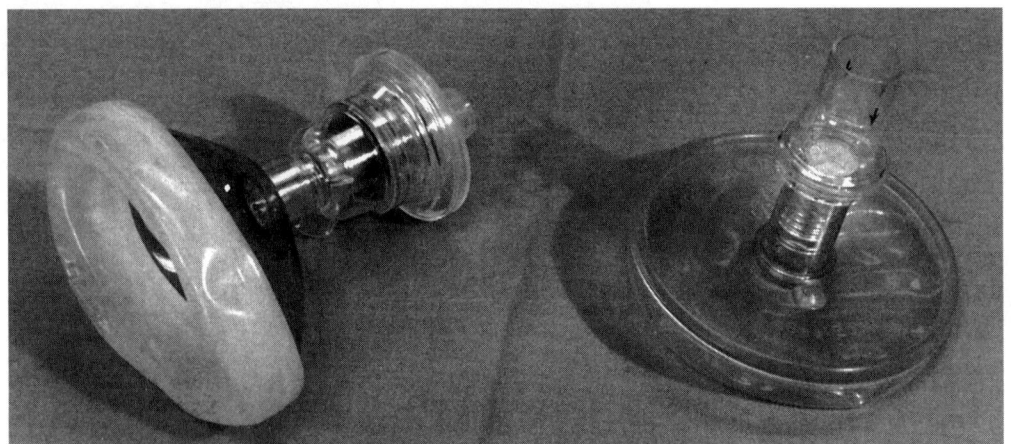

Figure 3-27   Two types of mouth-to-valve mask or pocket mask devices

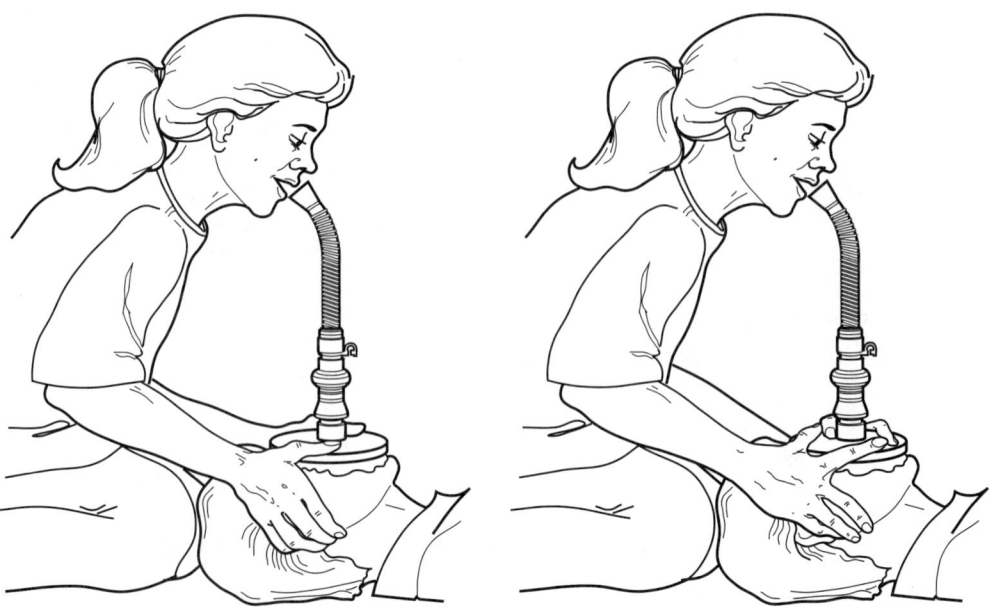

Figure 3-28   Two different ways to hold a mask to the patient's face to prevent an air leak when blowing into the mouth-to-valve mask unit

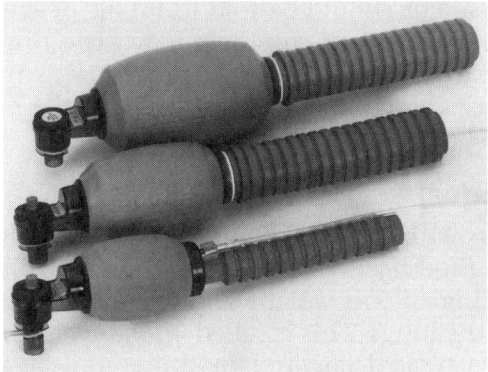

Figure 3-29 Three sizes of resuscitation bag: (*from the top*) adult, pediatric, and infant. An appropriately sized mask is connected to the valve at the left. Supplemental oxygen is added by tubing on the right side.

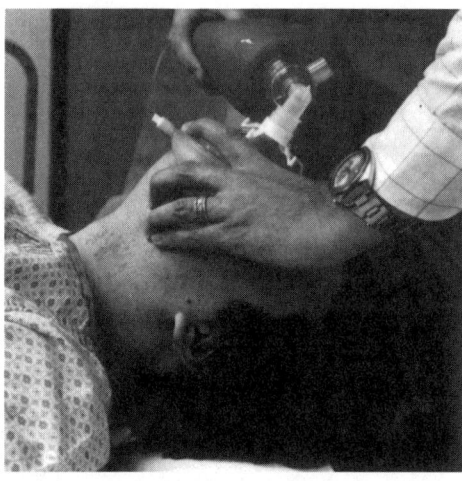

Figure 3-30 An adult being manually ventilated with a face mask and resuscitation bag

■ *electrical defibrillation:* *stopping fibrillation (quivering) of the heart by an electric device that applies electrical current through the electrodes on the chest wall*

units have outlets that connect to a CPR mask as well as an endotracheal or tracheostomy tube. Procedures for both ventilation devices are included later in this chapter and laboratory and clinical checkoff lists are provided in the Appendix. During a CPR attempt, you may also be expected to perform chest compressions, so be prepared to do so if the patient has no pulse. Additionally, you may be asked to get equipment such as an endotracheal tube, arterial blood gas kit, or tank of portable oxygen. During a CPR attempt, the resuscitation team is led by a physician and the RCP and RN have specific duties they have been specially trained for. **Electrical defibrillation** may be done to shock the patient's heart back to a normal rhythm. Be prepared to help any of the team members if possible.

▬▬ REMOVING PULMONARY SECRETIONS

Pulmonary secretions are removed in the following ways: cough and deep breathing exercises, oropharyngeal suctioning, deep tracheal suctioning, and bronchoscopy.

Cough and Deep Breathing Exercises

Cough and deep breathing exercises are among the simplest yet most important procedures that can be done to keep a patient's lungs working properly. Many bedridden patients do not sigh deeply as they normally would. This is especially true of patients who have had thoracic or abdominal surgery. Because of the postoperative pain, these patients do not want to inhale deeply and cough. For these reasons, many patients develop atelectasis and the resulting hypoxemia. Often the pulmonary secretions are not cleared normally and the foreign matter that they carry is not removed from the airways. Instead, bacteria multiply, leading to bronchitis and/or pneumonia.

It is very important to get patients out of bed and walking as quickly as possible so that their lungs expand more normally. The patient who cannot leave bed must be encouraged to frequently take deep breaths and cough. The deep breath sighs will help to prevent atelectasis and the cough will remove any airway secretions. The patient with postoperative abdominal or chest pain can be helped in two ways to do cough and deep breathing exercises. First, medication can be given as needed to decrease exercise-related pain. Second, a pillow can be used as a splint against the surgical wound. It can be held in place by the patient or you. The patient should be told to inhale deeply, hug the pillow against the incision, and cough. Your employer may expect that you can assist with cough and deep breathing exercises. This procedure is included later in this chapter and laboratory and clinical checkoff lists for the procedure are included in the Appendix.

Oropharyngeal Suctioning

Many patients with a stroke or other neurological injury lose the ability to swallow saliva or food normally. They may have it run out of the mouth. This can be embarrassing to the patient and family. Worse, the saliva or food may be inhaled into the lungs. This is called *aspiration* and may make the patient cough. Some of the aspirated saliva or food may not be coughed out completely and thus will stay within the patient's airways and lungs. This is a dangerous situation for two reasons. First, the saliva or food will plug the airways, decreasing the patient's oxygen level. Though not a common occurrence, aspirated food can completely obstruct the trachea and cause suffocation. Second, saliva or food that stays within the airways can cause a pulmonary infection.

Oropharyngeal suctioning is done to remove saliva or food from the patient's mouth by use of a suctioning tool and vacuum. A stiff, hollow plastic device called a *Yankauer* or *tonsil tip suction* is used, along with a rubber tube connected to a vacuum source, to suction out oral secretions or food (Figure 3-31). Use only as much suction pressure as needed. The RCP or RN should set the suction level and make any adjustments. It is usually safe to place the catheter tip into the patient's mouth between the cheek and gums. Apply suction only as long as needed. Be careful about placing the catheter tip in the back of the throat (oropharynx), because it may trigger the gag reflex. Failure to suction out anything could be from a disconnection of the tubing or from the suction system

Key Concept: *If the patient is making loud, abnormal breathing sounds from deep within the chest, get the RCP or RN immediately. The patient likely needs deep tracheal suctioning by the RCP or RN.*

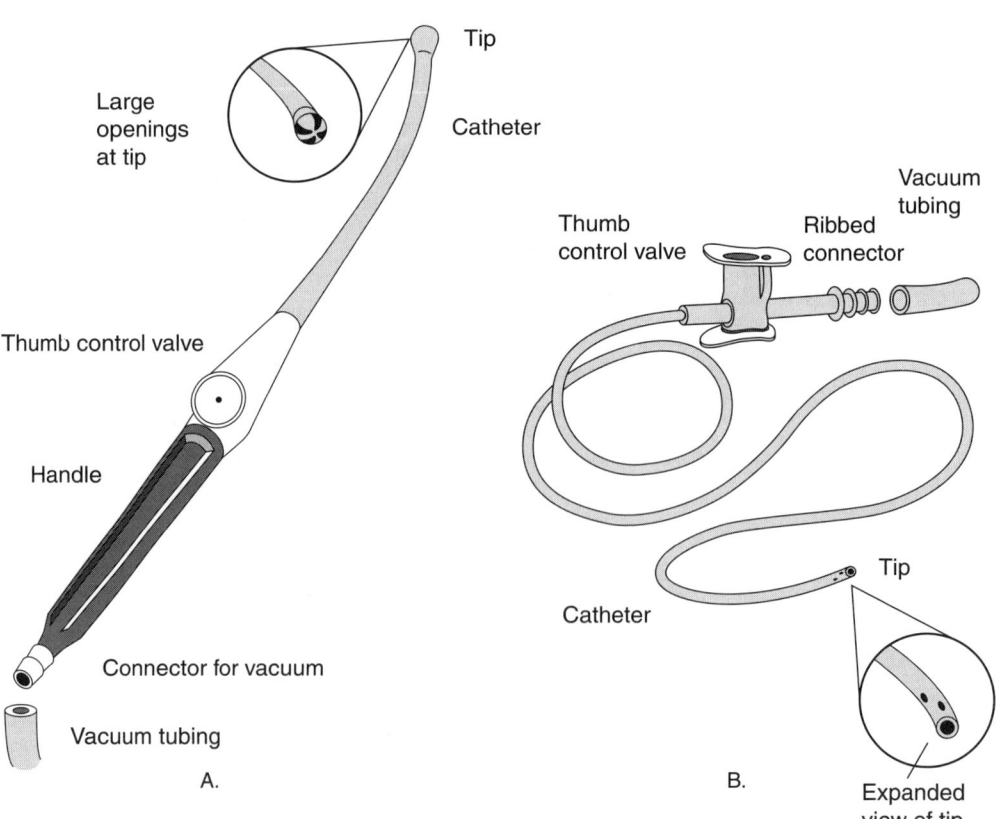

Figure 3-31   A. Features of a Yankauer suction catheter B. Features of a suction catheter with hollow tip and side holes

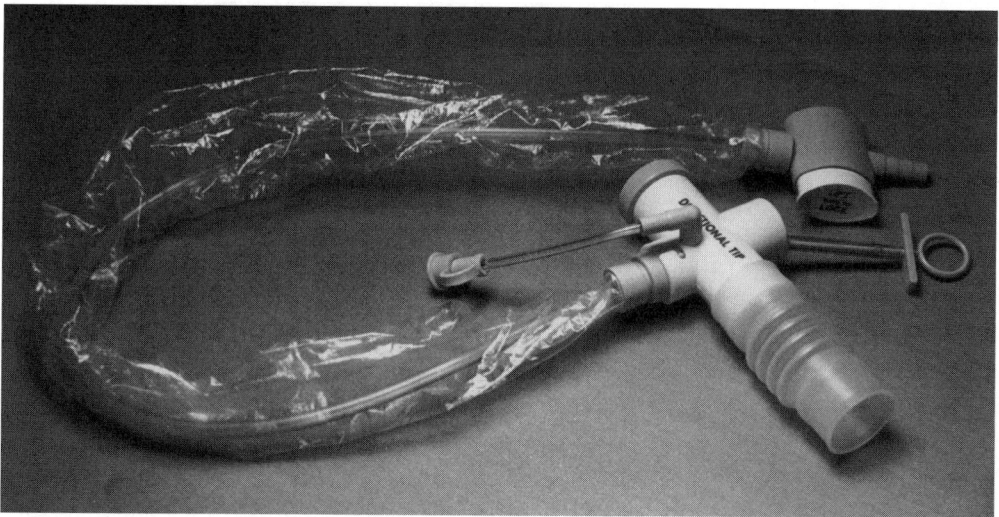

Figure 3-32 Trach Care Suction System, used with patients on a mechanical ventilator

not being turned on properly. Your employer may expect that you can assist with or perform oropharyngeal suctioning after proper training. A laboratory and clinical checkoff procedure for oropharyngeal suctioning is included in the Appendix. Remember, oropharyngeal suctioning will only remove saliva or food from the mouth. It will not remove any secretions from the lungs.

Deep Tracheal Suctioning

Deep tracheal suctioning, also called *endotracheal suctioning,* involves placing a long, flexible, hollow catheter into the patient's trachea. Endotracheal suctioning is done to remove secretions or food from the patient's trachea. The catheter is attached to rubber tubing that connects to the vacuum/suction source (Figures 3-31 and 3-32). Endotracheal suctioning is a sterile procedure and is usually performed only by an RCP, RN, or physician. The patient who has a tracheostomy tube or endotracheal tube will have the catheter advanced through it into the trachea. Other patients will have the catheter advanced through the nasal passage or a nasopharyngeal airway into the trachea. This procedure is called *nasotracheal suctioning.* You may be asked to assist in the following ways:

1. Getting the proper type of suction catheter.
2. Getting supplies such as sterile gloves, clean gloves, and sterile water-soluble lubricant.
3. Positioning the patient for suctioning as directed.
4. Monitoring the patient's pulse oximetry value and vital signs.

Bronchoscopy

This sophisticated instrument is a flexible, multi-channel catheter that can be guided into any of the patient's airways. The bronchoscope has a viewing channel through which the airways can be seen and a suction channel through which secretions can be suctioned or airway tissue samples taken. The bronchoscopy procedure is only performed by a physician. An RCP or RN usually assists in the procedure.

◼ POSTURAL DRAINAGE THERAPY

Postural drainage therapy involves placing patients into certain positions to help improve their cardiopulmonary condition. Frequently patients are positioned to keep the airway open. The patient who is comatose or under the influence of relaxing or pain-relieving medications may not be able to protect his or her airway. The tongue can block the upper airway, or oral secretions can fill the

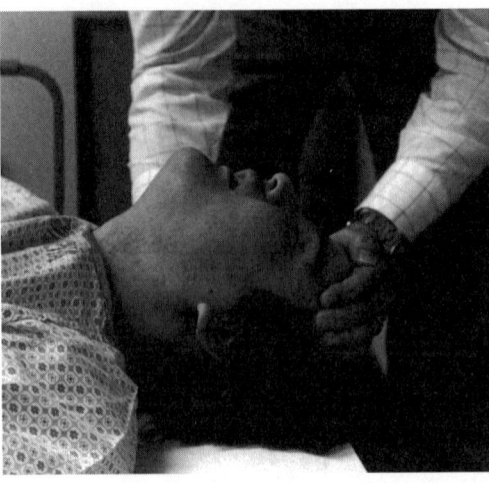

Figure 3-33 Patient with head tilted into the "sniffing position" to relieve upper airway obstruction

throat and be aspirated into the lungs. The upper airway can be kept open by placing the patient's head and neck into what is called the *sniffing position,* with the head hyperextended (Figure 3-33). In most patients, this will open the upper airway for normal breathing. Only the RCP, RN, or physician should place the patient into a sniffing position, because of the risk of a neck injury. It is also helpful to adjust the bed so that the patient's head is elevated and the knees are bent. You should continue to monitor the patient's breathing.

Atelectasis (collapsed alveoli) is a common problem in a patient who cannot get out of bed or turn himself or herself. Regular turning of the patient helps to prevent or treat atelectasis. Often a patient is rolled from side to back to other side to back on a timed schedule. These position changes are done to promote deeper breathing in alternating lungs. You may be needed to assist the RCP or RN in positioning the patient properly.

Postural Drainage with Percussion and Vibration

Postural drainage involves positioning the patient in specific ways to drain mucus from the bronchi that lead to the various lobes and segments of the lungs. The patient may at times be placed so that the head and chest are lower than the legs. Percussion and vibration involve gentle clapping and vibrating over the chest wall to loosen secretions for drainage. In most institutions the RCP performs these procedures; in other institutions the RCP or **physical therapist (PT)** may perform them. You may be expected to monitor the patient after the treatment is finished. Commonly the patient will continue to cough out loosened secretions after the RCP has left the room.

■■■ HYPERINFLATION THERAPY

All of the following procedures are done to open up the patient's alveoli to treat or prevent atelectasis: incentive spirometry, intermittent positive pressure breathing therapy, and continuous positive airway pressure.

Incentive Spirometry

The incentive spirometry procedure is done to encourage a patient to take in a deep breath. It is usually done along with cough and deep breathing exercises. Incentive spirometry is ordered by the physician either to treat existing atelectasis or to prevent its development. A number of incentive spirometry devices are available. Figures 3-34 and 3-35 show two different types.

The RCP should evaluate the patient, determine his or her inspired volume goal, coach the patient to properly perform incentive spirometry, and evaluate

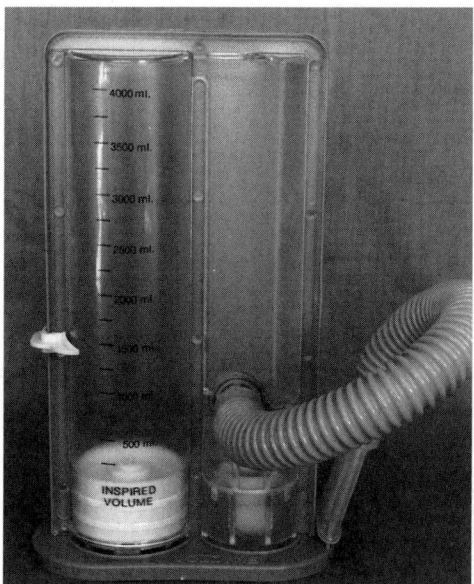

Figure 3-34 A Voldyne Volumetric Exerciser used in incentive spirometry. The inspired volume is noted in the left column.

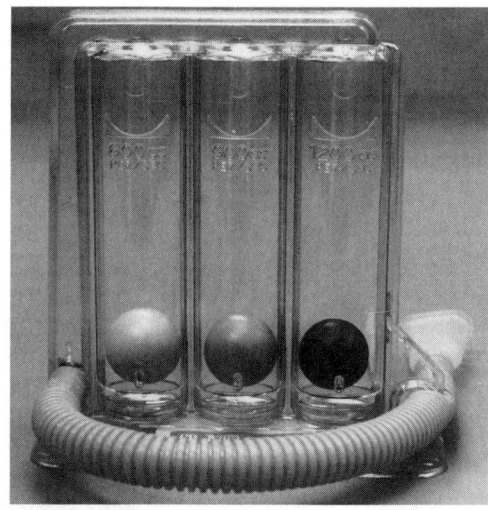

Figure 3-35 A Sherwood Medical Triflo device used in incentive spirometry. The inspired volume is based upon how many balls are lifted.

its results. When incentive spirometry is done properly, the patient inhales and holds as deep a breath as possible. The device measures the patient's inhaled volume. The goal is to reach the intended volume. After taking the deep breath, the patient holds it for a few seconds. This helps to prevent atelectasis and open up areas of collapsed alveoli. Incentive spirometry breathing should be done several times per hour while the patient is awake. The patient should cough after the procedure is completed.

Incentive spirometry is a safe procedure. However, patients who have had recent chest or abdominal surgery may complain of pain. Pain medication should help. The patient who takes too many deep breaths in a row may hyperventilate and blow off too much carbon dioxide. This may cause a temporary feeling of dizziness or tingling fingers. Tell the patient to relax and just breathe normally until he or she feels normal again. Depending on the institution, the RCP may continue to administer incentive spirometry, or the RN or you may be expected to continue the treatments. A procedure for incentive spirometry is included later in this chapter. Laboratory and clinical checkoff lists on the procedure are provided in the Appendix. Monitor the patient's breathing during and after the treatment. Report to the RCP or RN any problems, such as the patient not being able to reach the volume goal, pain, or hyperventilation. Record the volume the patient inhaled, how often he or she was able to do so, productive cough, and any complications.

Intermittent Positive Pressure Breathing Therapy

Patients who have atelectasis and cannot perform incentive spirometry, or need inhaled medications but cannot use an aerosol inhaler, are given intermittent positive pressure breathing (IPPB) therapy. It is given by a mechanical device powered by compressed air or oxygen. Figures 3-36 and 3-37 show two of the common IPPB machines and Figure 3-38 shows the IPPB breathing circuit that attaches to the machine. Only the RCP should be giving IPPB treatment. You may be asked to monitor the patient after the treatment and encourage coughing out any secretions.

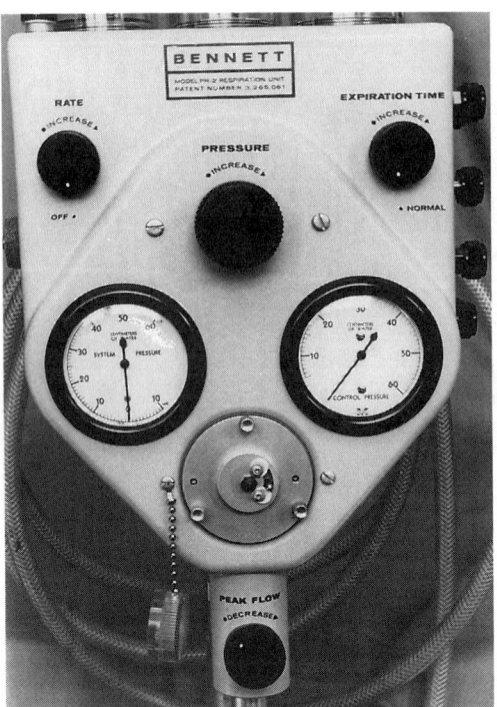

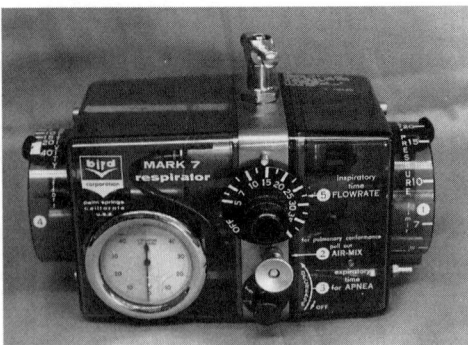

Figure 3-37 The front of a Bird MARK 7 machine used for intermittent positive pressure breathing treatments. The controls regulate the pressure sent to the patient and other factors in the treatment.

Figure 3-36 The front of a Bennett PR-2 machine used for intermittent positive pressure breathing treatments. The controls regulate the pressure sent to the patient and other factors in the treatment.

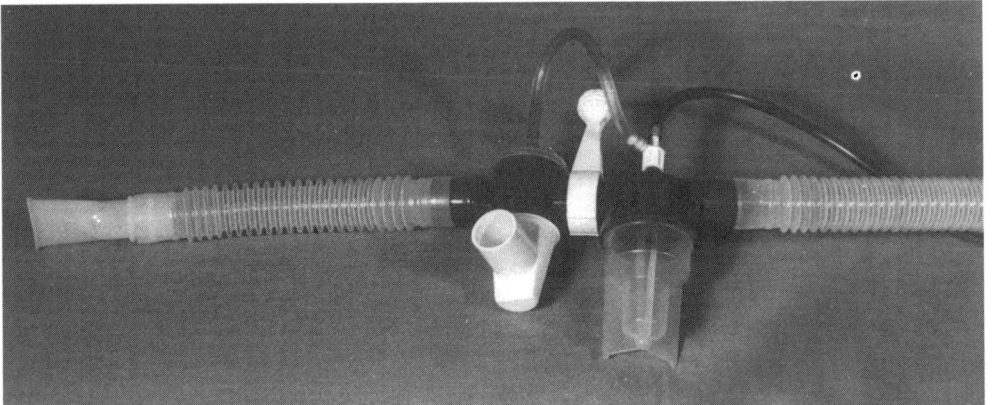

Figure 3-38 Breathing circuit used in an IPPB treatment, including the medication nebulizer and patient mouthpiece. The circuit is attached to either a Bennett or Bird IPPB machine.

■■■ Key Concept:

Contact the RCP or RN if an alarm is noted. Stay with the patient to make sure he or she is still able to breathe. Remove the CPAP device and resuscitate the patient who is not breathing. **■■■**

Continuous Positive Airway Pressure

Continuous positive airway pressure (CPAP) treatment involves a breathing circuit and nasal or face mask that applies continuous pressure to the patient's airway. CPAP is used to open up atelectatic areas or to keep the upper airway open in a patient with obstructive sleep apnea. The patient may be in the hospital to have the CPAP system set up and adjusted so that he or she can take it home and treat the sleep apnea problem. Only the RCP should be working with this equipment. Usually one or more audible and visual alarm systems are built into the CPAP system to warn of a malfunction.

▆▆ PHYSICIAN PROCEDURES

Bronchoscopy

Bronchoscopy is a special procedure undertaken to view the airways and remove secretions, as discussed earlier.

▆▆ Key Concept:
Report to the physician, RN, or RCP immediately if the patient coughs up any blood or complains of shortness of breath after the procedure. Stay with the patient until help arrives. ▆▆

Thoracentesis

This procedure involves a needle being placed through the chest wall and into the patient's pleural space. The physician can then remove air or any fluid (such as edema, blood, or pus) from the pleural space. Once the air or fluid is removed the lung should expand and the patient should be able to breathe more easily. The needle is then removed. An RN or RCP will usually assist with this procedure. You may be asked to help position the patient as needed and monitor the patient during and after the procedure.

Closed-Chest Drainage

For closed-chest drainage, the physician places a hollow rubber tube into the patient's pleural space. The other end of the tube is attached to a vacuum system that removes any air or fluid from the pleural space. The tube may stay in the patient for several days if needed. An RN or RCP usually assists with this procedure. You may be asked to help position the patient as needed and monitor the patient during and after the procedure.

▆▆ Key Concept:
Report to the physician, RN, or RCP immediately if the patient coughs up any blood, complains of shortness of breath after the procedure, or the vacuum system disconnects. Stay with the patient until help arrives. ▆▆

▆▆ MECHANICAL VENTILATION

A mechanical ventilator is a very sophisticated breathing machine with alarms, a humidification system, and a breathing circuit (Figure 3-39). It can provide a tidal volume with added oxygen a given number of times per minute to a

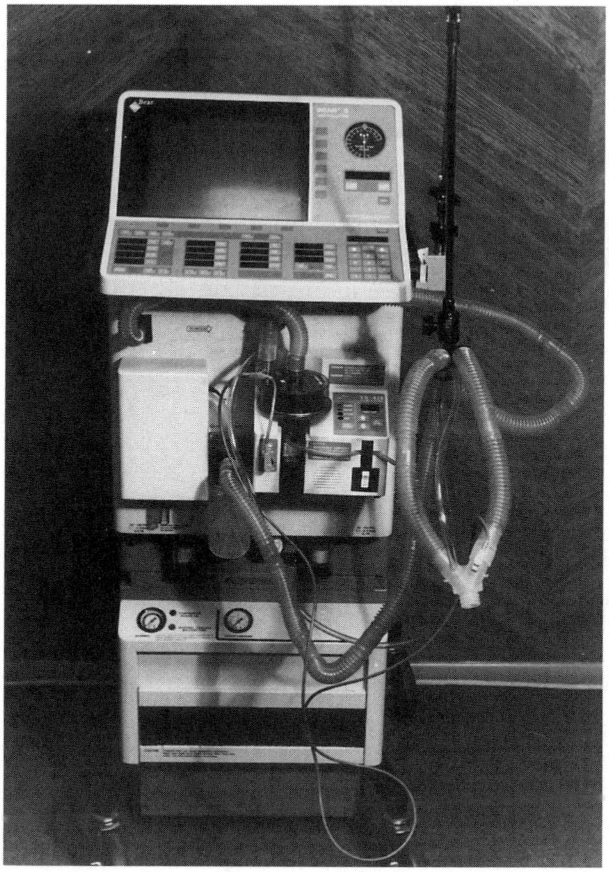

Figure 3-39 A BEAR 5 mechanical ventilator, assembled and ready to use. The breathing circuit delivers gas to the patient's endotracheal or tracheostomy tube. The controls regulate the oxygen percentage, tidal volume, respiratory rate, and other factors.

patient who is unable to breathe. The mechanical ventilator is also called a *ventilator, respirator,* or *life support system.* Patients who are very sick and cannot support their own breathing are mechanically ventilated. Often these patients are found in the intensive care unit. However, some patients may be stable enough to be maintained on a ventilator in an extended care facility or even at home. Examples of the types of patient conditions that require mechanical ventilation include, but are not limited to, pneumonia, emphysema, open heart surgery, lung surgery, **anesthesia,** and injury to the head, neck, chest, or abdomen.

A mechanical ventilator is operated by an RCP under the orders of a physician. The RN is also very involved in care of the ventilator-dependent patient. Many of the treatments discussed earlier are also used with these patients in the hope of correcting their problem(s). When a patient has recovered, he or she is gradually weaned off the ventilator. The endotracheal tube or tracheostomy tube can then usually be removed so that the patient breathes normally. You may help in the care of ventilator-dependent patients by performing oropharyngeal suctioning, positioning, general nurse assisting care, and basic patient monitoring. If an audible or visual alarm should go off, you should immediately call the RCP or RN. Stay with the patient and make sure he or she can still breathe. If the ventilator circuit is disconnected from the patient's endotracheal or tracheostomy tube, reconnect it. Inform the RCP or RN of this.

■ *anesthesia:* the absence of normal sensation, especially sensitivity to pain. Some anesthesia medications can temporarily cause shallow breathing or apnea

■■ **Key Concept:** *Call for help immediately if a ventilator alarm goes off. Stay with the patient until help arrives. Be prepared to use the resuscitation bag.* ■■

■■ PATIENT AND FAMILY EDUCATION

The physician, RN, and RCP are the primary patient educators. They will teach the patient and family about the patient's disease, its care, and any related equipment. You should be aware of these issues as well. There will be occasions when you need to reinforce something that was previously taught. If the patient is still unable to understand or perform a procedure, inform the individual who did the original teaching or someone from that department. They will then reinstruct the patient or family member.

■■ SPECIFIC RESPIRATORY CARE PROCEDURES FOR THE PATIENT CARE TECHNICIAN

The remainder of this chapter consists of cardiopulmonary procedures. Your institution may expect that you can perform some or all of them in patient care areas. These same procedures likely are also performed by members of the Respiratory Care Department. Depending on how your institution is organized, you will likely be taught to perform these procedures by members of the Respiratory Care Department. Members of the Nursing Department may also teach you these procedures. Remember that even though you may be taught to perform these procedures, you are not an expert on them. If you are unsure of any patient care activity you are performing, get an RCP or RN for assistance.

In preparing to be checked off on these procedures, it is recommended that you take the following steps:

■ Study the content of this text.

■ Look up the answers to the verbal questions in the laboratory and clinical checkoff lists that will be asked of you before you are permitted to attempt the procedure. The answers for the lab checkoff are included in the discussion of the topics in this chapter. Some of the clinical questions will require you to read the patient's chart or talk with your supervisor/ instructor or the RCP or RN to find the answers.

■ Assuming that there is an organized class to help you learn, understand the material that is presented to you. Each institution may have a different way of approaching the same procedure. You must be able to perform as expected in your institution and follow institutional policies.

- Practice the laboratory checkoff on the procedure with a partner who will act as the patient. Some of the procedures will also involve the use of life-like mannequins for practice. Practice how you will approach and what you will say to the patient as well as how you will perform the procedure. Practice writing down any charting that may have to be done.

- After passing the laboratory checkoff, practice the procedure (under the supervision of an instructor) on real patients. Practice talking to the patient, doing the procedure, and completing the charting.

- After passing the clinical checkoff on the procedure, remember that there is still much to learn. Many institutions will do a follow-up evaluation later to ensure that you are still able to safely perform the procedure.

PROCEDURE

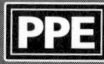

1 USE OF A RESUSCITATION BAG AND MASK DURING CPR

Introduction

A patient who is not breathing spontaneously must be artificially ventilated. The resuscitation bag is squeezed to deliver a volume of air or oxygen to the patient. The patient end of the bag can attach to a face mask or directly to the patient's endotracheal or tracheostomy tube. Both the resuscitation bag and face mask come in different sizes depending on the size of the patient. Supplemental oxygen is usually added to the bag with a reservoir. See Figure 3-29 for several different sizes of resuscitation bag and Figure 3-30 for a patient being ventilated with a resuscitation bag and mask.

Equipment Required

- appropriately sized resuscitation bag
- appropriately sized face mask to attach to the resuscitation bag
- oxygen tubing to connect the bag to an oxygen source
- oxygen flowmeter with tubing adapter
- oxygen source such as piped-in wall oxygen or an oxygen tank

Preparation

1. If needed, connect the face mask to the resuscitation bag.
2. Connect the oxygen tubing to the resuscitation bag gas inlet and the oxygen flowmeter.
3. Turn the flowmeter to the flow rate recommended by the manufacturer of the

resuscitation bag or as directed by the RCP, RN, or physician.

Precautions

Oxygen supports fire, so make sure there are no open flames near the flowmeter or bag.

Procedure

1. Put clean gloves on both hands. Institutional policy may also require you to put on a face mask and/or eye goggles.

    Rationale: *Standard precautions are followed to protect the caregiver and the patient.*

2. Select the proper resuscitation bag. Select the correct bag for the size of the patient. A bag that is too small will not deliver an adequate volume to the patient. A bag that is too large can overventilate a small patient and damage the lungs.

3. Select the additional equipment needed (flowmeter with tubing adapter, oxygen tubing, face mask). Although the patient can be ventilated with room air, supplemental oxygen is added as quickly as possible. If the patient is not intubated, a properly sized face mask must be obtained.

4. Connect bag, oxygen tubing, flowmeter, and face mask, if needed. All of these must be properly connected in order to ventilate the patient with supplemental oxygen.

5. Set the proper oxygen flow on the flowmeter. Ask the supervisor/instructor, RCP, or RN for the oxygen flow, or check the literature that

continues

PROCEDURE   1   *continued*

comes with the bag to find the oxygen flow in liters per minute that is recommended by the manufacturer. (Often a flow of 10 to 15 liters per minute is set for an adult bag. Less would be set on a smaller bag.)

6. Attach bag to patient's artificial airway, *or* attach bag and face mask to patient, as appropriate.

   The patient who has an endotracheal or tracheostomy tube can have the patient end of the bag directly attached to the tube. A face mask must be attached to the bag if the patient is not intubated.

7. Squeeze the bag at the appropriate rate. Typically an adult is ventilated at a rate of 12 breaths per minute—once every 5 seconds. A child is typically ventilated at a rate of 20 times per minute—once every 3 seconds.

8. Squeeze the bag to deliver an appropriate volume. Either one or two hands can be used to squeeze the bag to empty most of its gas. The patient's chest should be seen to rise as the bag is squeezed. Some resistance should be felt to the gas being forced into the patient's lungs.

   ▨▨ **Note:** *If the bag is squeezed and the patient's chest does not rise, something is wrong with the bag or the bag/mask attachment to the patient. Check what you are doing, the bag, the mask, or get help.* ▨▨

9. Monitor the patient's breathing, pulse, and appearance. The chest should be seen to rise with each squeeze of the bag. A carotid or femoral pulse should be checked for a heartbeat. Often a patient who is being adequately ventilated with a good pulse will return to normal color.

   ▨▨ **Rationale:** *If resuscitation efforts are effective, the patient should respond. If the patient has no pulse, chest compressions should be started.* ▨▨

10. Report observations to proper health care personnel. Tell the physician, RCP, or RN what you observed about the patient before and after the emergency occurred.

11. Chart as necessary (date, time, procedure, patient condition). It may be necessary to document these items if they are not charted by the RCP or RN.

12. After the procedure is completed, return the room to its normal condition and replace any used equipment or supplies.

    ▨▨ **Rationale:** *This is necessary in case the patient should again require emergency assistance.* ▨▨

Quality Assurance

Replace any equipment that fails. The failed item must be labeled and given to the RCP to be repaired or discarded. If an oxygen tank runs empty, it must be replaced with a full one.

Reporting and Interpreting Results

Inform a physician, RCP, or RN of what happened with the patient.

Documentation

As noted at step 11, you may need to document what happened with the patient. The charting must include the complete date, time of the incident and time of charting, the procedure performed, and your name and job title.

Patient Education

There is no patient education with this procedure.

2 USE OF A MOUTH-TO-VALVE MASK (POCKET MASK) DURING CPR

Introduction

A patient who is not breathing spontaneously must be artificially ventilated. The mouth-to-valve mask or pocket mask is used by the rescuer to ventilate the patient. Use of the mouth-to-valve mask prevents the spread of infection between the rescuer and patient. Some of the devices can have supplemental oxygen added to them. Make sure the mouth-to-valve mask fits the patient's face (see Figures 3-27 and 3-28).

Equipment Required

- mouth-to-valve mask, including face mask, one-way valve, and rescuer mouthpiece

- (if attachable) oxygen tubing to connect the mouth-to-valve mask to an oxygen source

- (if attachable) oxygen flowmeter with tubing adapter

- (if attachable) oxygen source, such as piped-in wall oxygen or oxygen tank

Preparation

1. Connect the face mask and mouthpiece to the one-way valve.

2. If attachable, connect the oxygen tubing to the adapter on the pocket mask and the oxygen flowmeter.

3. If attachable, turn on the flowmeter to the flow rate recommended by the manufacturer of the mouth-to-valve mask.

Precautions

Oxygen supports fire, so make sure there are no open flames near the flowmeter or pocket mask.

Procedure

1. Put clean gloves on both hands.

    Rationale: *Standard precautions are followed to protect the caregiver and the patient.*

2. Select the proper mouth-to-valve mask. Currently, only an adult size is available. If available, choose one that can have supplemental oxygen added.

3. Select additional equipment, if used (flowmeter with tubing adapter, oxygen

tubing). Although the patient can be ventilated by the rescuer's exhaled breath, supplemental oxygen should be added to the mask if possible.

4. Assemble the valve, mask, and mouthpiece. Make sure the device is assembled so that the rescuer's exhaled breath goes to the face mask.

5. Connect oxygen tubing and flowmeter to mask, if used. If supplemental oxygen can be added, an oxygen adapter will be located on the one-way valve or face mask. Attach the oxygen tubing to it. The other end of the oxygen tubing should be connected to the flowmeter and to the oxygen source.

6. Set the proper oxygen flow on the flowmeter, if used. Ask the supervisor/instructor, RCP, or RN for the oxygen flow, or check the literature that comes with the unit to find the oxygen flow in liters per minute that is recommended by the manufacturer.

7. Attach face mask to patient. Institutional policy may also require you to put on a face mask and/or eye goggles. An airtight seal is needed to ventilate the patient (see Figure 3-28).

8. Blow into the mouthpiece at an appropriate rate. Typically an adult is ventilated at a rate of 10 to 12 breaths per minute. A child is typically ventilated at a rate of 20 times per minute.

9. Blow into the mouthpiece to deliver an appropriate volume. Look at the patient's chest; the chest should rise as you blow into the mouthpiece. Some resistance should be felt to the gas being forced into the patient's lungs.

    Note: *If you blow into the device and the patient's chest does not rise, something is wrong with the device or the mask is not sealed on the patient's face. Check what you are doing, the device, the mask, or get help.*

10. Monitor the patient's breathing, pulse, and appearance. The chest should be seen to rise with each rescuer breath. A carotid or femoral

continues

pulse should be checked for heartbeat. Often a patient who is being adequately ventilated with a good pulse will return to normal color.

▄▄ **Rationale:** *If resuscitation efforts are effective, the patient should respond. If the patient has no pulse, chest compressions should be started.* ▄▄

11. Report observations to proper health care personnel. Tell the physician, RCP, or RN what you observed about the patient before and after the emergency occurred.

12. Chart as necessary (date, time, procedure, patient condition). It may be necessary to document these items if they are not charted by the RCP or RN.

13. After the procedure is completed, return the room to its normal condition and replace any used equipment or supplies.

▄▄ **Rationale:** *This is necessary in case the patient should again require emergency assistance.* ▄▄

Quality Assurance

Replace any equipment that fails. The failed item must be labeled and given to the RCP to be repaired or discarded. If an oxygen tank runs empty, it must be replaced with a full one.

Reporting and Interpreting Results

Inform a physician, RCP, or RN of what happened with the patient.

Documentation

As noted at step 12, you may need to document what happened with the patient. The charting must include the complete date, time of the incident and time of charting, the procedure performed, and your name and job title.

Patient Education

There is no patient education with this procedure.

PROCEDURE   PPE

3   PULSE OXIMETRY

Introduction

Pulse oximetry (SpO_2) is a relatively simple, noninvasive way to monitor a patient's oxygenation. It measures the level of saturation of the patient's hemoglobin with oxygen. The amount of saturation is given as a percentage (%). A variety of sensors are available that attach to a finger tip or toe, ear lobe, bridge of nose, forehead, or foot. The sensor is attached to the pulse oximeter. The patient's saturation, and usually a pulse rate, are displayed on the pulse oximeter. The device may also contain alarms that can be set for patient safety (see Figure 3-1).

The saturation percentage reported by the pulse oximeter should be reliable as long as the patient has good blood flow at the sensor site, does not have an elevated carbon monoxide level, does not have dark skin pigmentation, and (if a finger sensor is used) does not have on nail polish.

Equipment Required

▄▄ pulse oximeter unit
▄▄ sensor appropriate for the measurement site

Preparation

1. Make sure the measurement site has good blood flow.

2. Nail polish on the patient must be removed if a finger sensor is used.

3. A finger or toe sensor is recommended if the patient has dark skin pigmentation.

Precautions

1. Make sure the sensor is not wrapped so tightly that blood flow is cut off.

2. Do not use a pulse oximeter on a patient known or suspected of having carbon monoxide poisoning.

continues

Procedure

1. Confirm that the physician's order is current and complete, including a pulse oximetry goal, and if the patient is to use supplemental oxygen.

   Besides ordering that the patient's saturation be checked, the physician should order what he or she wants the minimum oxygen saturation to be. In most cases the minimum SpO_2 is kept at 90% to 92%. However, in different patients other values are targeted. It is also very important to make sure that the patient is breathing the ordered level of oxygen when the pulse oximetry value is measured.

2. Review the chart for current patient information. Confirm the ordered percentage of inhaled oxygen. Do not use pulse oximetry if the patient is suspected or known to have carbon monoxide poisoning.

3. Greet the patient, identify yourself, and state your purpose.

   Note: *It is always appropriate to greet the patient, identify yourself, and tell the patient why you are there.*

4. Check the patient's identity on his or her wristband. This will confirm that he or she is the correct patient for the procedure.

5. Make sure the oximeter sensor is properly placed on the patient. Adjust the equipment if needed.

   Place the sensor on the appropriate area as directed by the manufacturer. When the equipment is set up properly, you should be able to measure a strong pulse and an oxygen saturation value that corresponds with the patient's pulse.

6. Make sure the oxygen flow or percentage is set as ordered. Confirm in the patient's chart what oxygen system was ordered. Make sure it is working properly. Call the RCP to correct any problem or make any adjustments.

7. Identify a strong signal indicating a reliable pulse oximetry reading. Get help if a reliable signal cannot be obtained.

   Most pulse oximeters will give a numerical or other signal that the patient's pulse is being measured. This is necessary for the oxygen saturation to be measured accurately. Get the RCP if you cannot get a strong signal or you have any questions about the reliability of the measurements.

8. Note the patient's pulse oximetry value. Record the patient's saturation as a percentage (%). Some pulse oximeters will print out the information on a piece of paper for placement in the chart.

9. Note the patient's pulse rate, if the instrument gives it. (Most units will give a pulse rate.) Record the value in the chart if necessary.

10. Monitor the patient's breathing, pulse, and appearance. Note the patient's breathing rate and effort, pulse if not given by the oximeter, and general appearance and color. Get the RCP or RN if the patient's cardiopulmonary status has deteriorated or changed significantly.

11. Report observations to proper health care personnel.

12. Chart as necessary (date, time, procedure, patient condition). It may be necessary to document these items if they are not charted by the RCP or RN.

13. After the procedure is completed, return the room to its normal condition and replace any used equipment or supplies. The room should always be fully stocked so that the next health care worker will find any needed supplies where they are expected.

Quality Assurance

The patient should have been breathing the ordered amount of oxygen for at least 15 minutes before you take a pulse oximetry reading. Get help if you cannot obtain a reliable pulse oximetry reading.

Reporting and Interpreting Results

Depending on your institution, you may be expected to verbally report the pulse oximetry results to your supervisor or to record them in the patient's chart. Get the RCP or RN immediately if the patient's pulse oximetry value is less than the desired level ordered by the physician. The low reading could indicate hypoxemia.

continues

PROCEDURE **3** *continued*

Documentation

If your institution expects you to record information in the patient's chart, you should write at least the complete date, the patient's SpO_2 value, how much oxygen the patient was breathing, the time of measurement, and your name.

Patient Education

If supplemental oxygen is ordered for the patient, he or she should be told to keep it on at all times. Oxygen safety rules, such as not smoking, should be reinforced to the patient.

PROCEDURE

4 MAINTENANCE OF A NASAL CANNULA

Introduction

Hypoxemia is a serious condition that must be quickly corrected. A variety of oxygen masks and other devices are available to deliver a set supply of oxygen to the patient. A nasal cannula is a simple system that directs oxygen directly into the patient's nostrils. It can provide a moderate amount of oxygen and is used with patients who are in stable condition. It is important that the patient keep the cannula in place at all times. Removing it for even a few seconds can result in the patient's blood oxygen level dropping. See Figure 3-6 for a nasal cannula and Figure 3-7 for one properly placed on a patient.

Equipment Required

- nasal cannula of the proper size and style
- humidifier, if needed, with sterile water
- oxygen flowmeter
- oxygen tubing adapter to add to the flowmeter if a humidifier is not used
- oxygen source, such as piped-in wall oxygen or oxygen tank

Preparation

1. All of the required items of equipment may have to be gathered if the RCP or RN has not already done so.
2. The patient and family must be informed that the patient will be receiving oxygen.

Precautions

Oxygen supports fire, so the patient should not smoke and no open flames should be near the flowmeter or patient. Additionally, nothing that could create a spark should be near them.

Procedure

1. Confirm that the physician's order is current and complete. There should be a current order stating the use of a nasal cannula and its oxygen flow. The RCP or RN should have already set up the system as ordered.

2. Review the chart for current patient information. It is always important to keep current with your patient's condition. When supplemental oxygen is being used, look for information that relates to the patient's cardiopulmonary system.

3. Greet the patient, identify yourself, and state your purpose.
    It is always proper to act in a professional manner. Identify yourself and tell the patient that you are there to make sure the nasal cannula is working properly.

4. Confirm the patient's identity on his or her wristband.

5. Wash your hands. Put on protective devices such as gloves, etc., if indicated. Following standard precautions protects the patient and reassures him or her of your cleanliness.

6. Make sure the equipment is properly placed on the patient. Adjust the equipment if needed.
    Make sure that the two prongs on the cannula go into the patient's nostrils. The tubing on the cannula should wrap around

continues

the patient's ears properly. The non-patient end of the cannula must be connected to either the humidifier or the oxygen adapter on the flowmeter. There should be no kinks in the tubing.

Rationale: *If the cannula is not placed properly on the patient, the oxygen cannot be inhaled. Disconnected or kinked tubing will not deliver the oxygen.*

7. Make sure the oxygen flowmeter is set as ordered. Look at the flowmeter to make sure that the flow indicator shows the ordered flow of oxygen. If the flow is not as ordered, you or the RN must contact the RCP to adjust the flow.

Rationale: *Oxygen is a drug and must be given in the amount ordered.*

8. If a humidifier is in use, check that the water is above the marked minimum level. Any humidifier bottle will have minimum and maximum water levels marked on it. If the water level is below the minimum, the humidifier must be refilled or replaced. Notify the RCP of the low water level.

Note: *There are many types of humidifier bottles. Some are used until empty and others can be refilled with sterile water. The RCP will determine what to do with a low or empty humidifier bottle.*

9. If a humidifier is in use, check that the pressure relief valve is operating normally. When operating properly, a humidifier makes very little noise. If the oxygen tubing is pinched closed, a pressure relief valve will make a whistling or popping sound. Try to locate the pinch in the tubing and unkink it. The whistling or popping sound will stop when the oxygen is flowing again. Get the RCP if the humidifier is still making noise.

Rationale: *Tubing that is pinched will not deliver the oxygen.*

10. Reinforce to the patient the need to keep the nasal cannula in place at all times and to observe the oxygen safely rules, such as no smoking and no open flames or sparks.

Rationale: *Some patients (and family members) may not understand the importance of the patient's oxygen or the risk of fire associated with the use of supplemental oxygen.*

11. Monitor the patient's breathing, pulse, and appearance. If the patient's hypoxemia has been corrected, he or she should feel better and have a slower breathing and heart rate. The patient's color may return to normal. If a patient does not respond well to the use of supplemental oxygen, you should tell the RN or RCP.

12. Report observations to proper health care personnel. Tell the RCP or RN anything of importance that relates to the patient's use of supplemental oxygen or his or her cardiopulmonary condition.

13. Chart as necessary (date, time, procedure, patient condition). It may be necessary to document these items if they are not charted by the RCP or RN.

14. After the procedure is completed, return the room to its normal condition and replace any used equipment or supplies.

    Sterile water should be replaced as it is used. When you open a new bottle of sterile water, write the date and time on the label. Discard any unused portion in 24 hours or as dictated by your institution's policy.

Quality Assurance

Make sure the patient is receiving the proper, ordered flow of oxygen. Additionally, make sure that the equipment is working properly, that water is maintained within the humidifier bottle, and that the patient is wearing the nasal cannula correctly.

Reporting and Interpreting Results

Inform your supervisor or the RCP or RN how the patient is responding to the supplemental oxygen. Any complaint by the patient of continued shortness of breath should be reported.

Documentation

As noted in step 13, you may need to chart what happened with the patient. The charting must include the complete date, time of the equipment being checked, how the patient is tolerating the supplemental oxygen, and your name and job title.

Patient Education

As noted in step 10, the patient and family may need reinforcement about the purpose of supplemental oxygen and the need for the patient to wear the oxygen cannula at all times. Reiterate the ban on open flames or sparks.

PROCEDURE

5 MAINTENANCE OF AN AIR ENTRAINMENT MASK

Introduction

Hypoxemia is a serious condition that must be quickly corrected. A variety of oxygen masks and other devices are available to deliver a set supply of oxygen to the patient. An air entrainment mask is an oxygen delivery system that includes a face mask and a special attached tube on the bottom of the mask. The tube is adjustable to allow a certain amount of room air to be mixed (*entrained*) with the added oxygen. The air entrainment mask can be set to deliver several different oxygen percentages, typically ranging from 24% to 50%. It is important that the patient keep the mask in place at all times. Removing it for even a few seconds can result in the patient's blood oxygen level dropping. If the patient removes the oxygen mask for a short time to take a drink of water, blow his or her nose, etc., the mask must be put back on afterward. It is also very important that the patient and family do not adjust or play with the entrainment tube, as the oxygen percentage may be accidentally changed. See Figure 3-10 for an air entrainment mask and Figure 3-11 for one properly placed on a patient.

Equipment Required

- air entrainment mask of the proper size and style
- humidifier, if needed, with sterile water (usually a humidifier is not used)
- oxygen flowmeter
- oxygen tubing adapter to add to the flowmeter, if a humidifier is not used
- oxygen source, such as piped-in wall oxygen or oxygen tank

Preparation

1. All the items of required equipment may have to be gathered if the RCP or RN has not already done so.
2. The patient and family must be informed that he or she will be receiving oxygen.

Precautions

Oxygen supports fire, so no open flames (or smoking) should be near the flowmeter or patient.

Additionally, nothing that could create an open spark should be near them.

Procedure

1. Confirm that the physician's order is current and complete. There should be a current order stating the oxygen percentage to be delivered by the air entrainment mask. The RCP will set up the mask and determine the proper flow of oxygen to it.

2. Review the chart for current patient information. It is always important to keep current with your patient's condition. When supplemental oxygen is being used, look for information that relates to the patient's cardiopulmonary system.

3. Greet the patient, identify yourself, and state your purpose.

   It is always proper to act in a professional manner. Identify yourself and tell the patient that you are there to make sure the oxygen mask is working properly.

4. Confirm the patient's identity on his or her wristband.

5. Wash your hands. Following standard precautions protects the patient and reassures him or her of your cleanliness.

6. Make sure the equipment is properly placed on the patient. Adjust the equipment if needed.

   Make sure that the oxygen mask is properly covering the patient's nose and mouth. The elastic strap should go over the patient's ears and behind the head. The air entrainment tube must not be covered by the patient's bedding or anything else. The oxygen tubing must be connected to the mask and either the humidifier or the oxygen adapter on the flowmeter. There should be no kinks in the tubing.

   ■■ **Rationale:** *If the mask is not placed properly on the patient, the oxygen cannot be inhaled. The air entrainment tube must be open to room air to work properly. Disconnected or kinked tubing will not deliver the oxygen.* ■■

continues

7. Make sure the oxygen flowmeter is turned on; look at the flowmeter to make sure. With this oxygen delivery system, the flow rate will vary depending on the oxygen percent the patient needs. If the flow is turned off, you or the RN must get the RCP immediately.

   ▓▓ **Rationale:** *Oxygen is a drug and must be given in the amount ordered.* ▓▓

8. If a humidifier is in use, check that the water is above the marked minimum level. Any humidifier bottle will have minimum and maximum water levels marked on it. If the water level is below the minimum, the humidifier must be refilled or replaced. Notify the RCP of the low water level.

   ▓▓ **Note:** *There are many types of humidifier bottles. Some are used until empty and others can be refilled with sterile water. The RCP will determine what to do with a low or empty humidifier bottle.* ▓▓

9. If a humidifier is in use, check that the pressure relief valve is operating normally. When operating properly, a humidifier makes very little noise. If the oxygen tubing is pinched closed, a pressure relief valve will make a whistling sound. Try to locate the pinch in the tubing and unkink it. The whistling sound will stop when the oxygen is flowing again. Get the RCP if the humidifier is still whistling.

   ▓▓ **Rationale:** *Tubing that is pinched will not deliver the oxygen.* ▓▓

10. Reinforce to the patient the need to keep the oxygen mask in place at all times, to not adjust it or cover it up, and to observe the oxygen safety rules against open flames or sparks.

    ▓▓ **Rationale:** *Some patients (and family members) may not understand the importance of the patient's oxygen or the risk of fire associated with the use of supplemental oxygen.* ▓▓

    Additionally, tell the patient and family not to make any adjustment in the air entrainment tube and not to cover the air entrainment tube.

    ▓▓ **Rationale:** *Adjusting the setting on the air entrainment tube will change the oxygen percentage that the patient gets. This can be dangerous.* ▓▓

11. Monitor the patient's breathing, pulse, and appearance. If the patient's hypoxemia has been corrected, he or she should feel better and have a slower breathing and heart rate. The patient's color may return to normal. If a patient does not respond well to the use of supplemental oxygen, you should tell the RN or RCP.

12. Report observations to proper health care personnel. Tell the RCP or RN anything of importance that relates to the patient's use of supplemental oxygen or his or her cardiopulmonary condition.

13. Chart as necessary (date, time, procedure, patient condition). It may be necessary to document these items if they are not charted by the RCP or RN.

14. After the procedure is completed, return the room to its normal condition and replace any used equipment or supplies.

    Sterile water should be replaced as it is used. When you open a new bottle of sterile water, write the date and time on the label. Discard any unused portion in 24 hours or as dictated by your institution's policy.

Quality Assurance

Make sure the flowmeter is running and that the patient is wearing the oxygen mask correctly. Additionally, if a humidifier is in use, make sure that it is not whistling or popping and that the water is above the minimum level.

Reporting and Interpreting Results

Inform the RCP or RN how the patient is responding to the supplemental oxygen. Any complaint by the patient of continued shortness of breath should be reported.

Documentation

As noted in step 12, you may need to chart what happened with the patient. The charting must include the complete date, time of the equipment being checked, how the patient is tolerating the supplemental oxygen, and your name and job title.

Patient Education

As noted in step 10, the patient and family may need reinforcement about the purpose of supplemental oxygen and the need for the patient to wear the oxygen equipment at all times. Reiterate the ban on open flames or sparks.

PROCEDURE

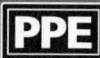

6 | MAINTENANCE OF A SIMPLE OXYGEN MASK

Introduction

Hypoxemia is a serious condition that must be quickly corrected. A variety of oxygen masks and other devices are available to deliver a set supply of oxygen to the patient. A simple oxygen mask and its attached oxygen tubing direct moderate amounts of oxygen to the patient's nose and mouth. The amount of oxygen given depends on the oxygen flow that is set. The simple oxygen mask is used with patients who are in stable condition. It is important that the patient keep the oxygen mask on at all times. Removing it for even a few seconds can result in the patient's blood oxygen level dropping. If the patient removes the mask for a short time to take a drink of water, blow his or her nose, etc., the mask must be put back on afterward. See Figure 3-8 for a simple oxygen mask and Figure 3-9 for one properly placed on a patient.

Equipment Required

- simple oxygen mask of the proper size and style
- humidifier, if needed, with sterile water
- oxygen flowmeter
- oxygen tubing adapter to add to the flowmeter, if a humidifier is not used
- oxygen source, such as piped-in wall oxygen or oxygen tank

Preparation

1. All of the items listed of required equipment may have to be gathered if the RCP or RN has not already done so.
2. The patient and family must be informed that he or she will be receiving oxygen.

Precautions

Oxygen supports fire, so no open flames should be near the flowmeter or patient. Additionally, nothing that could create an open spark should be near them.

Procedure

1. Confirm that the physician's order is current and complete. There should be a current order stating the use of a simple oxygen mask and its oxygen flow. The RCP or RN should have already set up the system as ordered.

2. Review the chart for current patient information. It is always important to keep current with your patient's condition. When supplemental oxygen is being used, look for information that relates to the patient's cardiopulmonary system.

3. Greet the patient, identify yourself, and state your purpose.

    It is always proper to act in a professional manner. Identify yourself and tell the patient that you are there to make sure the oxygen mask is working properly.

4. Confirm the patient's identity on his or her wristband.

5. Wash your hands. Following standard precautions protects the patient and reassures him or her of your cleanliness.

6. Make sure the equipment is properly placed on the patient. Adjust the equipment if needed.

    Make sure that the oxygen mask is properly covering the patient's nose and mouth. The elastic strap should go over the patient's ears and behind the head. The oxygen tubing must be connected to the mask and either the humidifier or the oxygen adapter on the flowmeter. There should be no kinks in the tubing.

    ▰▰ **Rationale:** *If the mask is not placed properly on the patient, the oxygen cannot be inhaled. Disconnected or kinked tubing will not deliver the oxygen.* ▰▰

7. Make sure the oxygen flowmeter is turned on; look at the flowmeter to make sure. With this oxygen delivery system, the flow rate will vary depending on the oxygen percent the patient needs. If the flow is turned off, you or the RN must get the RCP immediately.

    ▰▰ **Rationale:** *Oxygen is a drug and must be given in the amount ordered.* ▰▰

continues

8. If a humidifier is in use, check that the water is above the marked minimum level. Any humidifier bottle will have minimum and maximum water levels marked on it. If the water level is below the minimum, the humidifier must be refilled or replaced. Notify the RCP of the low water level.

   ▓▓ **Note:** *There are many types of humidifier bottles. Some are used until empty and others can be refilled with sterile water. The RCP will determine what to do with a low or empty humidifier bottle.* ▓▓

9. If a humidifier is in use, check that the pressure relief valve is operating normally. When operating properly, a humidifier makes very little noise. If the oxygen tubing is pinched closed, a pressure relief valve will make a whistling sound. Try to locate the pinch in the tubing and unkink it. The whistling sound will stop when the oxygen is flowing again. Get the RCP if the humidifier is still whistling.

   ▓▓ **Rationale:** *Tubing that is pinched will not deliver the oxygen.* ▓▓

10. Reinforce to the patient the need to keep the oxygen mask in place at all times and to observe the oxygen safety rules against open flames or sparks.

    ▓▓ **Rationale:** *Some patients (and family members) may not understand the importance of the patient's oxygen or the risk of fire associated with the use of supplemental oxygen.* ▓▓

11. Monitor the patient's breathing, pulse, and appearance. If the patient's hypoxemia has been corrected, he or she should feel better and have a slower breathing and heart rate. The patient's color may return to normal. If a patient does not respond well to the use of supplemental oxygen, you should tell the RN or RCP.

12. Report observations to proper health care personnel. Tell the RCP or RN anything of importance that relates to the patient's use of supplemental oxygen or his or her cardiopulmonary condition.

13. Chart as necessary (date, time, procedure, patient condition). It may be necessary to document these items if they are not charted by the RCP or RN.

14. After the procedure is completed, return the room to its normal condition and replace any used equipment or supplies.

    Sterile water should be replaced as it is used. When you open a new bottle of sterile water, write the date and time on the label. Discard any unused portion in 24 hours or as dictated by your institution's policy.

Quality Assurance

Make sure the patient is receiving the proper, ordered flow of oxygen. Additionally, make sure that the equipment is working properly, that adequate water is in the humidifier bottle, and that the patient is wearing the oxygen mask correctly.

Reporting and Interpreting Results

Inform the RCP or RN how the patient is responding to the supplemental oxygen. Any complaint by the patient of continued shortness of breath should be reported.

Documentation

As noted in step 13, you may need to chart what happened with the patient. The charting must include the complete date, time of the equipment being checked, how the patient is tolerating the supplemental oxygen, and your name and job title.

Patient Education

As noted in step 10, the patient and family may need reinforcement about the purpose of supplemental oxygen and the need for the patient to wear the oxygen equipment at all times. Reiterate the ban on open flames or sparks.

PROCEDURE

7 MAINTENANCE OF A NONREBREATHER MASK

Introduction

Hypoxemia is a serious condition that must be quickly corrected. A variety of oxygen masks and other devices are available to deliver a set supply of oxygen to the patient. A nonrebreather mask is a system that includes a face mask, attached oxygen reservoir bag, and oxygen tubing. It can provide a high percentage of oxygen and is used with patients who are very hypoxic. It is critically important that the patient keep the oxygen mask in place at all times. Removing it for even a few seconds can result in the patient's blood oxygen level dropping very low. If the patient removes the oxygen mask for a short time to take a drink of water, blow his or her nose, etc., the mask must be put back on afterward. See Figure 3-12 for a nonrebreather mask and Figure 3-13 for one properly placed on a patient.

Equipment Required

- nonrebreather mask of the proper size and style
- humidifier, if needed, with sterile water
- oxygen flowmeter
- oxygen tubing adapter to add to the flowmeter, if a humidifier is not used
- oxygen source, such as piped-in wall oxygen or oxygen tank

Preparation

1. All of the items of required equipment may have to be gathered if the RCP or RN has not already done so.
2. The patient and family must be informed that he or she will be receiving oxygen.

Precautions

Oxygen supports fire, so no open flames should be near the flowmeter or patient. Additionally, nothing that could create an open spark should be near them.

Procedure

1. Confirm that the physician's order is current and complete. There should be a current order stating the use of a nonrebreather mask; the oxygen flow is determined by the RCP.

The RCP or RN should have already set up the system as ordered.

2. Review the chart for current patient information. It is always important to keep current with your patient's condition. When supplemental oxygen is being used, look for information that relates to the patient's cardiopulmonary system.

3. Greet the patient, identify yourself, and state your purpose.

   It is always proper to act in a professional manner. Identify yourself and tell the patient that you are there to make sure the oxygen mask is working properly.

4. Confirm the patient's identity on his or her wristband.

5. Wash your hands. Following standard precautions protects the patient and reassures him or her of your cleanliness.

6. Make sure the equipment is properly placed on the patient. Adjust the equipment if needed.

   Make sure that the oxygen mask is properly covering the patient's nose and mouth. The elastic strap should go over the patient's ears and behind the head. The oxygen reservoir bag attached to the mask must not be covered with bedding.

7. Make sure the oxygen flowmeter is turned on; look at the flowmeter to make sure. With this oxygen delivery system, the flow rate will vary depending on the patient's breathing depth and rate. The bag must stay at least half full as the patient inhales. You or the RN must call the RCP if the bag collapses too much during inspiration. The oxygen tubing must be connected to the mask and either the humidifier or the oxygen adapter on the flowmeter. There should be no kinks in the tubing.

   Rationale: *If the mask is not placed properly on the patient, the oxygen cannot be inhaled. The reservoir bag must stay inflated to give the patient as much oxygen as possible.*

continues

Disconnected or kinked tubing will not deliver the oxygen. ▪▪▪

If the flow is turned off, you or the RN must get the RCP immediately.

▪▪▪ **Rationale:** *Oxygen is a drug and must be given in the amount ordered.* ▪▪▪

8. If a humidifier is in use, check that the water level is above the marked minimum level. Any humidifier bottle will have minimum and maximum water levels marked on it. If the water level is below the minimum, the humidifier must be refilled or replaced. Notify the RCP of the low water level.

   ▪▪▪ **Note:** *There are many types of humidifier bottles. Some are used until empty and others can be refilled with sterile water. The RCP will determine what to do with a low or empty humidifier bottle.* ▪▪▪

9. If a humidifier is in use, check that the pressure relief valve is operating normally. When operating properly, a humidifier makes very little noise. If the oxygen tubing is pinched closed, a pressure relief valve will make a whistling or popping sound. Try to locate the pinch in the tubing and unkink it. The whistling or popping sound will stop when the oxygen is flowing again. Get the RCP if the humidifier is still making noise.

   ▪▪▪ **Rationale:** *Tubing that is pinched will not deliver the oxygen.* ▪▪▪

10. Reinforce to the patient the need to keep the oxygen mask in place at all times and to observe the oxygen safety rules against open flames or sparks.

    ▪▪▪ **Rationale:** *Some patients (and family members) may not understand the importance of the patient's oxygen or the risk of fire associated with the use of supplemental oxygen.* ▪▪▪

11. Monitor the patient's breathing, pulse, and appearance. If the patient's hypoxemia has been corrected, he or she should feel better and have a slower breathing and heart rate. The patient's color may return to normal. If a patient does not respond well to the use of supplemental oxygen, you should tell the RN or RCP.

12. Report observations to proper health care personnel. Tell the RCP or RN anything of importance that relates to the patient's use of supplemental oxygen or his or her cardiopulmonary condition.

13. Chart as necessary (date, time, procedure, patient condition). It may be necessary to document these items if they are not charted by the RCP or RN.

14. After the procedure is completed, return the room to its normal condition and replace any used equipment or supplies.

    Sterile water should be replaced as it is used. When you open a new bottle of sterile water, write the date and time on the label. Discard any unused portion in 24 hours or as dictated by your institution's policy.

Quality Assurance

Make sure the patient is receiving the proper, ordered flow of oxygen. Additionally, make sure that the equipment is working properly, that water within the humidifier bottle is above the minimum level, that the patient is wearing the oxygen mask correctly, and that the reservoir bag stays inflated.

Reporting and Interpreting Results

Inform the RCP or RN how the patient is responding to the supplemental oxygen. Any complaint by the patient of continued shortness of breath should be reported.

Documentation

As noted in step 13, you may need to chart what happened with the patient. The charting must include the complete date, time of the equipment being checked, how the patient is tolerating the supplemental oxygen, and your name and job title.

Patient Education

As noted in step 10, the patient and family may need reinforcement about the purpose of supplemental oxygen and the need for the patient to wear the oxygen equipment at all times. Reiterate the ban on open flames, smoking, or sparks.

8 INCENTIVE SPIROMETRY

Introduction

Incentive spirometry is done to encourage a patient to take deep breaths. Cough and deep breathing exercises are then performed. These two things are done either to prevent a patient from developing atelectasis (collapsed alveoli) or to treat a patient who has atelectasis. These patients often also have excessive secretions that must be coughed out. Atelectasis can be caused by shallow breathing in a postoperative chest or abdominal patient or a bedridden patient. Opening up atelectatic areas of the lungs should help to improve the patient's oxygen level. Figures 3-34 and 3-35 show two types of incentive spirometer devices.

Equipment Required

- incentive spirometer device
- facial tissue to cough into
- if needed, a pillow to support the surgical wound

Preparation

1. The patient must be alert and cooperative.
2. It is best if the patient sits up in a chair or on the edge of the bed; minimally, raise the head of the bed as high as possible.
3. Make sure the incentive spirometer is put together properly.
4. The patient should be able to reach the incentive spirometer and the facial tissue.

Precautions

There are no dangers in performing incentive spirometry. However, recent postoperative patients may complain of incisional pain. Pain medication should help with this. A pillow can be used to support the wound when coughing. Dizziness or tingling fingers can result from hyperventilating if the patient inhales deeply too many times in a row. The patient should relax and not do incentive spirometry until he or she feels normal again.

Procedure

1. Confirm that the physician's order is current and complete. There should be a current order stating how often the patient is to perform incentive spirometry.

2. Review the chart for current patient information. It is always important to keep current with your patient's condition. There must be a pulmonary problem that can be treated by incentive spirometry. The RCP will determine the inhaled volume goal for the patient.

3. Greet the patient, identify yourself, and state your purpose.

   It is always proper to act in a professional manner. Identify yourself and tell the patient that you are there to help him or her with the incentive spirometry treatment.

4. Confirm the patient's identity on his or her wristband.

5. Wash your hands. Following standard precautions protects the patient and reassures him or her of your cleanliness.

6. Make sure the equipment is properly set up for the patient. Adjust the equipment if needed.

   The mouthpiece, tubing, and incentive spirometer must be set up correctly. Adjust them if necessary so that the patient can easily use the unit.

7. If a target volume or target flow has been chosen, set it for the patient. Some incentive spirometers have a marker for the patient's volume goal or flow goal. Make sure it is set properly or adjust the marker to the goal.

8. Ask the patient to exhale normally and then inhale as deeply as possible and hold the breath for 3 to 4 seconds.

   The deep breath and breath hold are needed for the prevention or treatment of atelectasis. If the patient cannot properly perform the treatment, it will not be helpful.

   ▆▆ **Rationale:** *Atelectasis is treated by taking as deep a breath as possible and holding the breath for several seconds.* ▆▆

9. Note the patient's inhaled volume and breath hold time. Observe if the patient can inhale the volume set for his or her goal. Count how many seconds the patient can hold in the deep breath.

continues

PROCEDURE **8** *continued*

▣ **Rationale:** *If the patient cannot take in a deep breath and hold it, the atelectasis will not be treated.* ▣

10. Encourage the patient to cough deeply. Taking a deep breath and coughing will open up the lungs and clear any secretions.

▣ **Rationale:** *Secretions must be removed for the lungs to work properly.* ▣

11. Encourage the patient to perform a proper incentive spirometry breath the number of times per hour that the physician has ordered. The awake and alert patient should be told to perform incentive spirometry as ordered even if the RCP, RN, or you are not available to help.

12. Monitor the patient's breathing, pulse, and appearance before, during, and after the treatment. If areas of atelectasis are opened up, the patient's oxygen level should increase. He or she should feel better and have a slower breathing and heart rate. The patient's color may return to normal. If the patient does not respond well to the treatment, you should tell your supervisor, the RN, or RCP.

13. Report observations to proper health care personnel. Tell the RCP or RN anything of importance that relates to the patient's treatment or his or her cardiopulmonary condition.

14. Chart as necessary (date, time, procedure, patient condition). It may be necessary to document these items if they are not charted by the RCP or RN.

15. After the procedure is completed, return the room to its normal condition and replace any used equipment or supplies. Restock facial tissue or a pillow if one is used.

Quality Assurance

Observe if the patient is able to reach the volume goal and how often. If the patient is unable to perform incentive spirometry, the RCP or RN must be notified.

Reporting and Interpreting Results

Inform the RCP or RN how the patient is responding to the treatment, volume reached, frequency of deep breathing, and productivity of the cough. Any complaint by the patient should be reported.

Documentation

As noted in step 14, you may need to chart what happened with the patient. The charting must include the complete date, time the procedure was performed, how the patient tolerated the procedure, and your name and job title.

Patient Education

Reinforce to the patient and family, as needed, the importance of performing incentive spirometry. Reinforce the need to perform cough and deep breathing exercises.

PROCEDURE

9 **COUGH AND DEEP BREATHING EXERCISES**

Introduction

Cough and deep breathing exercises are very important to prevent or treat atelectasis and to clear pulmonary secretions. Patients who do not breathe deeply are likely to develop atelectasis or worse pulmonary problems, such as bronchitis or pneumonia. These may be patients who recently had chest or abdominal surgery and are in pain, or they may be bedridden and unable to breathe deeply. Often, an incentive spirometry treatment is given before the patient is encouraged to cough and deep breathe.

Equipment Required

- ▪ facial tissue to cough into
- ▪ if needed, a pillow to support the surgical wound

continues

- sputum sample container, if a sample is ordered

Preparation

1. The patient must be alert and cooperative.

2. It is best if the patient sits up in a chair or on the edge of the bed; minimally, raise the head of the bed as high as possible.

Precautions

There are no risks with the cough and deep breathing procedure. Pain may be felt by a patient who recently had surgery. The RN may give the patient something for pain so that he or she can cooperate completely.

Procedure Steps

1. Confirm that the physician's order is current and complete. There should be a current order for the patient to cough and deep breathe. An order may also be written to get a sample of sputum from the patient for laboratory testing.

2. Review the chart for current patient information. It is always important to keep current with your patient's condition. There must be a pulmonary problem that can be treated by the cough and deep breathing exercise.

3. Greet the patient, identify yourself, and state your purpose.

   It is always proper to act in a professional manner. Identify yourself and tell the patient that you are there to help him or her to cough and deep breathe.

4. Confirm the patient's identity on his or her wristband.

5. Wash your hands. Following standard precautions protects the patient and reassures him or her of your cleanliness.

6. Get a pillow or blanket to support an incision, if needed; either may be used. The patient should be able to wrap his or her arms around the pillow or folded blanket. Some patients may prefer to support the incision with their hands only.

7. Position a bedbound patient with head elevated for comfort, bent knees, and hands or pillow supporting a chest or abdominal incision. Position the patient in as upright a position as possible. The pillow or blanket

should not be held tightly to the body while inhaling.

8. Have the patient breathe two or three times in through the nose and out through the mouth. Several deep breaths help to open up areas of atelectasis. The surgical patient also gets used to the level of discomfort that comes from taking a deep breath.

9. Have the patient inhale as much as possible and perform as strong a cough as possible. The deeper the patient inhales, the more volume he or she has to cough out with. A strong cough will blow out any secretions. The surgical patient may hold the pillow or blanket tightly *only* when coughing out.

10. Have the patient cough out any sputum that is produced into a tissue so that you can see it. Swallowing sputum can upset the stomach of some patients. If a sputum sample is needed for laboratory tests, the patient should cough into the collection jar. Give the sputum sample to the RN or RCP.

11. Note the amount, color, odor, and consistency of the sputum.

    People usually do not cough up sputum. Patients with pulmonary problems will have a productive cough. If a patient coughs into a container, the amount can be measured. If a patient coughs into a facial tissue and throws it away, estimate the amount of sputum as small, medium, or large. Normal sputum is clear or white in color and without odor. Patients with pulmonary problems may have sputum that is yellow, green, brown, or bright red in color, and the sputum will be sticky and not very watery. The RCP may have the patient inhale medications that make the sputum easier to cough out. Note if the patient can cough out the secretions more easily after a breathing treatment. Be prepared to report your observations to the RCP or RN.

    ■■ **Rationale:** *The amount, color, and consistency of the patient's sputum is important, as it relates to how the patient is responding to treatment.* ■■

    ■■ **Key Concept:** *Get help immediately if the patient begins to cough out bright red sputum— it may be blood.* ■■

12. Monitor the patient's breathing, pulse, and appearance before, during, and after a cough

continues

and deep breathing exercise. If the patient coughs out any sputum, his or her breathing may be easier afterward. Oxygenation may improve and the patient's color may return to normal.

13. Report observations to proper health care personnel. Tell the RCP or RN anything of importance that relates to the patient's cough and deep breathing exercise. Note any change in amount, color, odor, or consistency of the patient's sputum.

14. Chart as necessary (date, time, procedure, patient condition). It may be necessary to document these items if they are not charted by the RCP or RN.

15. After the procedure is completed, return the patient to his or her former position and the room to its normal condition. The patient may be more comfortable back in bed or with the head in a lower position. Return anything that was moved, such as the overbed table.

Quality Assurance

Make sure that the patient gives a good effort in performing a cough and deep breathing exercise.

Tell the RN or RCP if the patient cannot perform the treatment.

Reporting and Interpreting Results

Inform the RCP or RN how the patient responded to the treatment. Any change in patient effort or amount, color, odor, or consistency of sputum should be reported. Tell your supervisor, the RCP, or RN if a sputum sample was obtained.

Documentation

As noted in step 14, you may need to chart what happened with the patient. The charting must include the complete date, time of the treatment, how the patient performed, and the results of the patient's effort. Chart if a sputum sample was obtained.

Patient Education

Reinforce to the patient the need to cough and deep breathe as the doctor has ordered to keep the lungs clear.

PROCEDURE   PPE

10 CHANGING A PORTABLE "E" TYPE TANK OF OXYGEN

Introduction

A portable tank of oxygen is needed whenever a patient receiving supplemental oxygen must be moved to another area of the facility. An "E" size tank of oxygen is typically used for patient transport because it is small and light enough to be lifted. When a tank has less than 500 psi (pounds per square inch) of pressure, it is considered empty. The regulator that controls the gas pressure and flow of oxygen from the tank must be removed from the empty tank and placed on a new "E" tank. Because the new tank contains pure oxygen under high pressure, the procedure must be done correctly to be safe. Figure 3-4 shows an "E" type tank of oxygen and Figure 3-5 shows an "E" tank regulator.

Equipment Required

- new "E" tank of oxygen
- regulator for an "E" tank of oxygen
- oxygen tank wrench
- new plastic O-ring washer from the new oxygen tank

Preparation

Move the old and new tanks of oxygen to a place away from any open flames and where they will not be knocked over.

Precautions

1. Oxygen tanks should not be stored near open flame, electrical appliances, or where anyone would smoke.

continues

PROCEDURE 10 *continued*

2. All oxygen tanks must be kept secured so that they will not be knocked over.

Procedure

1. Slowly turn on the old tank to check its pressure and confirm that it is empty. (It is acceptable to turn on the tank and state the pressure at which a tank should be changed.)

Refer to Figure 3-40 as you read this. The top, stainless steel part of the tank is called the *post*. The regulator attaches to it. Inside the post is a *direct-acting valve* that allows the oxygen to be released in a controlled manner. The topmost part of the direct-acting valve is a small metal bar called the *valve stem* or *control valve*. When the valve stem is turned counterclockwise, the direct-acting valve is opened and gas will leave the tank. Turning the valve stem clockwise turns off the gas flow. A *tank wrench* has one or two rectangular slit openings that fit over the valve stem so the tank can be turned on and off.

The *yoke connector* of the regulator attaches the regulator to the post of the tank.

Place the small slit opening of the tank wrench over the valve stem on the top of the oxygen tank. Slowly turn the tank wrench counterclockwise, opening up the tank. The pressure from the gas will be seen on the pressure gauge on the regulator. Remember, a full tank has at least 2,000 psi and an empty tank has less than 500 psi. Note the tank pressure. Assuming that it is less than 500 psi, the tank is empty and the rest of the procedure may be followed.

2. Turn off the tank by turning the tank wrench clockwise. The pressure will still be seen on the gauge.

3. Turn on the flowmeter to bleed the pressure out of the regulator (let the gas within the regulator leak out). In the example shown in Figure 3-5, the knob is turned clockwise. The

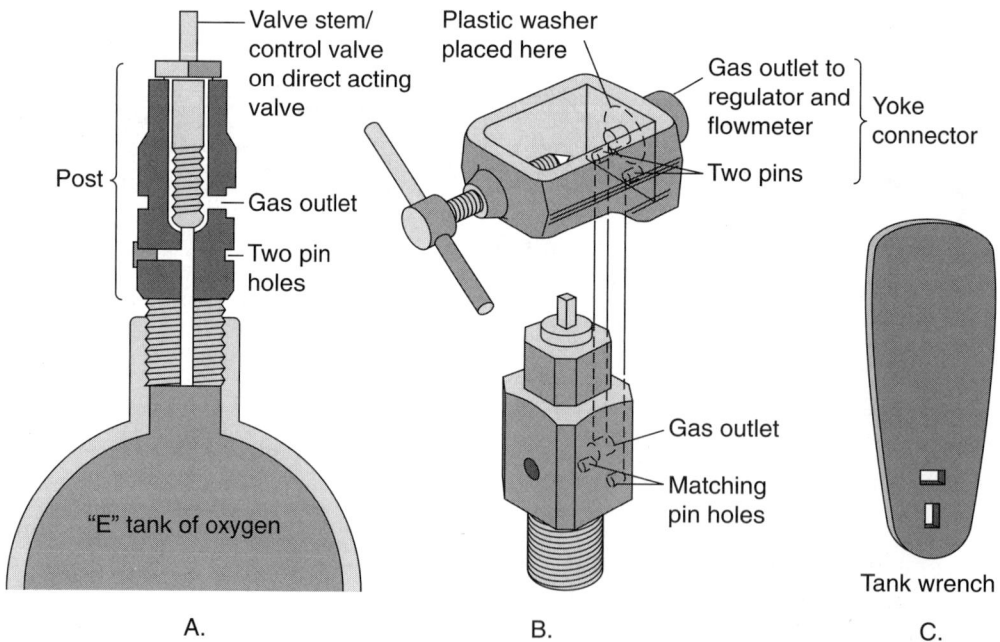

A.   B.   C.

Figure 3-40 A. A cross-section through the stem and direct-acting valve of an "E" tank. Details include the valve stem or control valve to control gas flow, the gas outlet, and the pin inserts where the yoke pins insert. B. Three-dimensional view of how a yoke connector attaches to the stem of an "E" tank. Details include the yoke connector, the gas outlet that attaches to the regulator (not shown), two pins that insert into the matching hole on the stem, and the gas outlet on the stem that matches to the gas outlet on the yoke and regulator. C. A tank wrench that connects to the valve stem so that the valve can be opened or closed.

continues

pressure gauge will drop down to a pressure of zero.

▨▨ **Note:** *Not all regulators are of this type. It is important to practice with the regulators used in your institution.* ▨▨

4. Turn off the flowmeter. In the example shown in Figure 3-5, the knob is turned counterclockwise. Other regulators may operate differently.

5. Remove the regulator from the tank. The yoke handle has two long, thin spokes for gripping. Turn the yoke handle counterclockwise to loosen the regulator from the post of the tank. The two pins on the yoke fit into the two matching holes on the post of the tank.

6. Remove and discard the old plastic washer from the regulator. The gas outlet for oxygen flow from the post of the tank is near the two pin holes. The matching gas outlet on the regulator is near the two pins on the yoke. A plastic O-ring washer is used to seal the opening between the post and the regulator. Remove and discard the old O-ring.

7. Label the tank as EMPTY; tape or tie an EMPTY sign on the old tank. Remember that it still contains some pure oxygen under pressure, so it must be stored safely.

8. Select a replacement tank by confirming that the adhesive label states it contains oxygen and that the tank is painted green in color.

▨▨ **Rationale:** *You must make sure the new tank is oxygen. Other tanks of other medical gases are also found in the hospital.* ▨▨

9. Remove the plastic protective covering from the post of the new tank.

10. Place the new plastic washer from the protective covering on the regulator. The new O-ring washer is placed on the yoke where the oxygen will enter the regulator from the gas outlet of the tank.

▨▨ **Rationale:** *The new washer will prevent an oxygen leak between the regulator and the tank when they are put together.* ▨▨

11. **Slowly** turn on the tank to "crack" it and blow any dust from the oxygen outlet. Put the small slit opening of the tank wrench over the valve stem of the new tank. Slowly turn the wrench counterclockwise to let some of the

oxygen leak out. Opening the tank too much will generate a LOUD sound of gas escaping. Turn off the tank to prevent further leakage.

12. Place and tighten the regulator onto the new tank. Place the yoke over the post so that the two yoke pins fit into the matching holes on the post. The O-ring washer on the yoke will line up with the oxygen outlet on the post. Turn the crank on the yoke clockwise so that the tip of it fits into the hole on the post. Tighten the crank.

13. Slowly turn on the tank and make sure there is no leak around the regulator. Tighten the regulator if needed. With the tank wrench over the valve stem, slowly turn the wrench counterclockwise to open up the tank. Gas will enter the regulator and pressure will be seen on the gauge. If oxygen is heard and/or felt to be leaking between the post and the yoke, tighten the crank until the leak stops. If the leak does not stop, turn off the tank, turn the crank counterclockwise to loosen the regulator for removal, and start over. Follow the preceding steps again and make sure that the O-ring washer is properly placed.

14. Note the pressure in the tank to confirm that it is full (about 2,000 psi). Look at the pressure gauge to determine the pressure in the tank. If needed, make a note of the pressure.

15. Turn off the tank by turning the tank wrench clockwise. This will turn off the oxygen tank to prevent waste.

16. Turn on the flowmeter to bleed the pressure from the regulator and let the oxygen within the regulator leak out. The pressure within the regulator will drop to zero.

17. Turn off the flowmeter so that oxygen does not rush out the next time the tank is turned on.

18. Put the tank in a secure place (tank cart, tank rack on wheelchair or transport gurney, or chained to wall). The tank should be stored so that it cannot be knocked over. There should not be open flames or sparks in the area where it is stored.

Quality Assurance

These steps must be carefully followed so that high-pressure oxygen does not leak out. By itself, an oxygen leak is not dangerous. However,

continues

increased oxygen in an area is a risk if there is an open flame. Additionally, wasting oxygen from the tank is expensive.

Reporting and Interpreting Results

Note the pressure within the new tank so that staff members know it is full.

Documentation

If needed, chart the date and time that you replaced the empty tank. Note the pressure within the new tank. Label the old tank as EMPTY.

Patient Education

Not applicable.

PROCEDURE

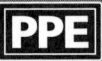

11 PREPARING A PORTABLE "E" TYPE TANK OF OXYGEN FOR PATIENT TRANSPORT

Introduction

Patients who need supplemental oxygen should never be without it. When a patient on supplemental oxygen needs to be transported from his or her room to another part of the facility, a portable "E" tank of oxygen is needed.

Note: *This procedure should not be attempted until after Procedure 10 has been completed.*

Equipment Required

- "E" tank of oxygen with a gauge pressure of at least 500 psi
- tank wrench

Preparation

Tell the patient that he or she needs to be moved for a test or procedure and that you are going to set up an oxygen tank.

Precautions

Follow all oxygen safety rules, including supporting the tank to prevent its being knocked over and keeping the tank away from open flames, smoking, and sparks.

Procedure

1. Confirm that the patient will need a portable oxygen tank for transportation. An order must be written for the patient to be transported for a test or procedure. If the patient is using supplemental oxygen, a portable oxygen system must go with him or her.

2. Greet the patient, identify yourself, and state your purpose.

   It is always proper to act in a professional manner. Identify yourself and tell the patient that you are there to set up an oxygen tank so that he or she can keep the oxygen system while being moved.

3. Confirm the patient's identity on his or her wristband.

4. Find out the type of oxygen delivery system the patient is using. This can be done by checking the order in the chart, looking at the system on the patient, or talking with the RCP.

5. Find out the oxygen flow that will be needed. The patient's oxygen flow should be the same on the "E" tank flowmeter as it is on the room flowmeter.

6. Find out if a humidifier is being used with the oxygen delivery system by looking at the patient's oxygen system in the room.

7. Slowly turn on the tank to make sure it is full enough for the transport. (It must have at least 500 psi.) Use the tank wrench to slowly turn the valve stem on the "E" tank in a counterclockwise direction. This will let the oxygen enter the regulator. Look at the pressure gauge to see the pressure within the tank.

   Rationale: *The tank is turned on slowly so that the pressure will not build up in the regulator too quickly.*

continues

The tank must have at least 500 psi to be used. A tank with less than 500 psi is considered empty.

▓▓ **Rationale:** *A tank that has less than 500 psi may run out completely while the patient is away from his or her room.* ▓▓

8. If a humidifier is needed, unscrew it (with the oxygen delivery system) from the patient's room oxygen flowmeter and screw it onto the flowmeter on the oxygen tank.

    There are two basic types of humidification systems. Figure 3-16 shows a bubble-type humidifier that connects to small-bore oxygen tubing. Figure 3-17 shows a large-volume nebulizer that connects to large-bore tubing. There are many different types of units, of several different styles. In all cases, the threaded connector on top can be unscrewed from the wall flowmeter. The unit can then be screwed onto the flowmeter on the regulator on the "E" tank. Make sure the connection is tight. The oxygen tubing and mask should be kept intact.

9. If no humidifier is needed, unscrew the oxygen tubing adapter (with the oxygen delivery system) from the room oxygen flowmeter and screw the oxygen tubing adapter onto the flowmeter on the oxygen tank.

    Some oxygen masks do not use a humidifier of any type. These systems all use small-bore tubing that is pushed onto an oxygen tubing adapter that has been screwed onto a wall flowmeter. To transfer this system, unscrew the oxygen tubing adapter from the wall flowmeter. Then screw the adapter onto the flowmeter on the regulator on the "E" tank. Make sure the connection is tight. The oxygen tubing and mask should be kept intact.

10. Turn on the tank's flowmeter to the needed oxygen flow. Turn off the room oxygen flowmeter. The RCP or RN will usually turn on the patient's oxygen through the "E" tank. If you have been approved to do so, you may turn on the flowmeter on the "E" tank to the same flow as the wall flowmeter.

11. Make sure the patient's oxygen delivery system is operating normally.

Refer to earlier discussions on the various types of oxygen masks and delivery systems. It is extremely important that the patient receive the same amount of supplemental oxygen on the portable system as he or she was getting before. If you are unsure, ask the RCP or RN to check the system.

12. Keep the oxygen tank in a vertical position if a humidifier is used. All humidifiers must be kept upright or the water will spill out.

13. Monitor the patient's breathing, pulse, and appearance. If the patient is getting supplemental oxygen as he or she is supposed to, there should not be any change in vital signs or appearance. If there is a problem, the patient's breathing, pulse, and appearance may change. Get the RCP or RN if the patient appears to be having difficulty.

14. Report observations to proper health care personnel. Tell the RCP or RN anything of importance that relates to the patient's use of supplemental oxygen or his or her cardiopulmonary condition.

15. Chart as necessary (date, time, procedure, patient condition). It may be necessary to document these items if they are not charted by the RCP or RN.

16. After the procedure is completed, return the patient to his or her former position and the room to its normal condition.

    After the patient is brought back to the room, make sure that he or she is put back in bed or a chair as necessary. The oxygen system must be switched from the "E" tank back to the wall oxygen flowmeter. Again, make sure that the patient is getting the same amount of supplemental oxygen now as before. Get the RCP or RN to be sure of this.

Quality Assurance

The patient must not be allowed to become hypoxic. Get the RCP or RN if there is any problem with the oxygen system.

Reporting and Interpreting Results

Inform the RCP or RN how the patient is responding to the supplemental oxygen. Any complaint by the patient of shortness of breath or other symptoms must be reported.

continues

PROCEDURE **11** *continued*

Documentation

Depending on your institution, you may or may not need to chart that the patient was transported with a supplemental oxygen system.

Client Education

Make sure the patient understands that he or she will still be getting the oxygen that is needed during the trip.

PROCEDURE

12 OROPHARYNGEAL SUCTIONING

Introduction

Oropharyngeal suctioning involves the removal of saliva, food, vomitus, and so forth from a patient's oral cavity. This procedure is done to help keep the upper airway clear.

Equipment Required

- electrically powered suctioning machine or wall vacuum suctioning system
- rubber tubing connected to the suctioning source
- Yankauer suction catheter (see Figure 3-31)
- clean latex gloves, goggles, and/or mask, depending on institutional policy
- bottle of sterile water or saline to rinse the catheter and tubing

Preparation

1. Assemble the suctioning source, rubber tubing, and Yankauer suction catheter.
2. Turn on the suctioning source.
3. Put gloves on both hands.
4. Tell the patient you are going to suction out his or her mouth.

Precautions

1. Avoid touching the back of the oral pharynx with the Yankauer device, as it may stimulate the gag reflex and cause vomiting.
2. Oropharyngeal suctioning may result in gagging, coughing, or vomiting reflexes.

Procedure

1. Confirm that the physician's order is current and complete. There should be a current order stating that the patient may have oropharyngeal suctioning done at given times or as needed.
2. Review the chart for current patient information. It is always important to keep current with your patient's condition. You should know why the patient needs oropharyngeal suctioning (for example, the patient had a stroke).
3. Greet the patient, identify yourself, and state your purpose.
   It is always proper to act in a professional manner. Identify yourself and tell the patient that you are there to clear out his or her mouth.
4. Confirm the patient's identity on his or her wristband.
5. Wash your hands or put on clean gloves, goggles, and mask according to your unit's policy. Protect yourself from possible contamination as necessary.

   ▪▪▪ **Rationale:** *Some patients may have an infection of the oral cavity that you would want to protect yourself against.* ▪▪▪

6. Gather and assemble the equipment, if needed. The suctioning system must be operating properly. One end of the suction tubing must be connected to the suctioning system. The other end of the suction tubing must be connected to the Yankauer suction catheter.
7. Turn on the suction unit. Adjust the pressure, if needed, to the level set by unit policy.

continues

PROCEDURE   12   *continued*

Practice with your suctioning system is needed for this step. There are several types of systems that operate differently. You should know how to turn your system on and off. The supervisor, RN, or RCP will determine and set the level of vacuum that can be used. If you have been approved to do so, you may be allowed to adjust the vacuum level.

8. Position the patient properly for suctioning. A patient can be suctioned in any position if necessary. However, if not contraindicated, raising the patient's head or turning the patient on a side may make his or her breathing easier. Ask the RN if the patient has any limits on positioning before suctioning.

9. Suction the oropharynx of the patient to remove secretions. The Yankauer catheter tip can be placed into the space between the cheek and teeth or gums where saliva will pool. This can be done to either or both sides. Avoid touching the back of the oropharynx with the catheter tip. Cover the thumb control valve to suction out the mouth contents. It is recommended that you do not suction for more than 5 seconds at a time.

10. Rinse the suction tip and tubing in a cup of sterile water or saline solution. After suctioning, remove the catheter from the patient's mouth. Place the catheter tip in the sterile water or saline cup and apply suction. Suction up the water or saline until the catheter is cleaned out.

11. Repeat steps 9 and 10 as needed. Suctioning may be repeated as necessary until the patient's mouth is cleared of saliva and other matter. It is recommended that suctioning not be applied for more than 5 seconds at a time. Let the patient rest between suctioning efforts.

12. Note the amount, color, odor, and consistency of the secretions. Look at the suction collection jar to see how much was suctioned from the patient. If you suspect that blood or vomitus is present, get the RN or RCP immediately.

13. Monitor the patient's breathing, pulse, and appearance before, during, and after the suctioning. Get help immediately if the patient is having difficulty breathing.

14. Report observations to proper health care personnel. Tell the RN or RCP anything of importance that relates to the patient's cardiopulmonary condition.

15. Chart as necessary (date, time, procedure, patient condition). It may be necessary to document these items if they are not charted by the RN or RCP.

16. After the procedure is completed, return the patient to his or her former position and the room to its normal condition. Put the patient in a comfortable position where he or she can breathe easily. Turn off the suctioning system. Discard your gloves and other personal protective equipment in the way prescribed by your institution. Wash your hands.

Quality Assurance

Make sure the equipment is set up and operating properly. Use only the vacuum level set by the RN or RCP unless you have been approved to make an adjustment. Use careful technique so as to not harm the patient.

Reporting and Interpreting Results

Inform your supervisor or the RN or RCP what was suctioned from the patient and how he or she tolerated the procedure.

Documentation

As noted in step 15, you may need to chart what was done with the patient. The charting must include the complete date, time of the procedure, results of the procedure, how the patient tolerated it, and your name and job title.

Patient Education

If the patient is conscious, tell him or her to use the nurse call button when suctioning needs to be done again. The family can also be told to call this way or to get you, the RN, or RCP when suctioning needs to be done again.

REVIEW QUESTIONS

Multiple Choice Questions

1. When a patient needs to be mechanically ventilated, what type of artificial airway is used?
   a. Endotracheal tube
   b. Oropharyngeal airway
   c. Nasopharyngeal airway
   d. Bronchoscopy tube

2. Your patient has an order to receive an aerosolized medication. What is your responsibility?
   a. Prepare the medication.
   b. Give the medication.
   c. Monitor the patient's breathing after the treatment is over.
   d. Chart the patient's response to the treatment in the chart.

3. A patient is positioned in bed in certain ways to do all of the following *except:*
   a. Prevent atelectasis.
   b. Prevent anemia.
   c. Maintain an open upper airway.

4. Halfway through an incentive spirometry treatment, your patient complains of dizziness and tingling fingers. What would you do?
   a. Call the nurse for help.
   b. Ask the nurse to give the patient a pain medication.
   c. Stop the treatment and tell the patient to breathe normally.
   d. Continue the treatment until completed and chart the patient's complaint.

5. Twenty minutes after a thoracentesis treatment, your patient coughs up blood. What would you do?
   a. Get a sputum cup to collect a blood sample.
   b. Call the nurse for help and stay with the patient.
   c. Get a blood gas sampling kit to collect a blood sample.
   d. Tell the patient not to cough so hard.
   e. Delay the next incentive spirometry treatment.

6. While turning a patient during a bed bath, the mechanical ventilator circuit pulls off his tracheostomy tube. What is the first thing that you should do?
   a. Call the nurse for help.
   b. Call the respiratory care practitioner for help.
   c. Reconnect the circuit to the tracheostomy tube.
   d. Ventilate the patient with the manual resuscitation bag.

7. A pulse oximeter measurement is done to determine the amount of what gas in a patient?
   a. Oxygen
   b. Nitrogen
   c. Water vapor
   d. Carbon dioxide
   e. Helium

8. All of the following can be used to help treat a patient with atelectasis *except:*
   a. Intermittent positive pressure breathing (IPPB).
   b. Cough and deep breathing exercises.
   c. Incentive spirometry.
   d. Pulmonary function test.

9. To make sure that a tank of gas contains oxygen, what should you do?
   1. Check the tank label.   a. 1, 2
   2. Make sure the tank is painted blue.   b. 3, 4
   3. Make sure the tank is painted green.   c. 2, 4
   4. Check the regulator on the tank.   d. 1, 3

10. Your patient is wearing a venturi mask. He says that he is cold and pulls the blankets up tight to his neck and covers over the tube at the bottom of the mask. What would you do?
    a. Get him another blanket.
    b. Uncover the tube and tuck the blanket underneath it.
    c. Turn up the oxygen flow.
    d. Change the air entrainment on the tube to increase the oxygen percentage.

11. All of the following can result in an abnormal finger pulse oximeter reading *except:*
    a. Dark skin pigmentation.
    b. Carbon monoxide poisoning.
    c. Normal blood pressure.
    d. Bright lights in the room.
    e. Dark fingernail polish.

12. Hypoxemia can be caused by all of the following *except:*
    a. Heart failure.
    b. Increased carbon dioxide level.
    c. Shallow breathing.
    d. Increased shunt from a pulmonary embolism.
    e. Cyanide poisoning.

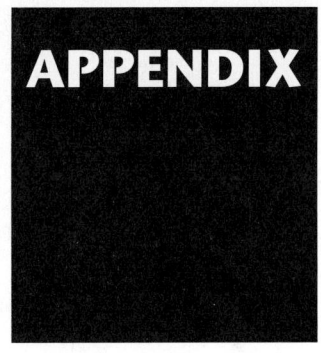

Procedure Checklists

PROCEDURE 1 CHECKLIST
USE OF A RESUSCITATION BAG AND MASK DURING CPR

Verbal questions that must be answered correctly before starting the procedure:

1. Identify when this equipment would be needed.
2. Identify the equipment needed for adult or pediatric patients.
3. Describe why supplemental oxygen is used.
4. Identify how to clear any obstruction from the equipment.

LABORATORY checkoff on the procedure.

DC	DI	NA	
___	___	___	1. Put clean gloves on both hands; and mask and goggles as needed.
___	___	___	2. Select the proper resuscitation bag.
___	___	___	3. Select the additional equipment needed (flowmeter with tubing adapter, oxygen tubing, face mask).
___	___	___	4. Connect bag, oxygen tubing, flowmeter and face mask, if needed.
___	___	___	5. Set the proper oxygen flow on the flowmeter.
___	___	___	6. Attach bag to patient's artificial airway, if appropriate. Attach bag and face mask to patient, if appropriate.
___	___	___	7. Squeeze the bag at the appropriate rate.
___	___	___	8. Squeeze the bag to deliver an appropriate volume.
___	___	___	9. Monitor the patient's breathing, pulse, and appearance.
___	___	___	10. Report observations to proper health care personnel.
___	___	___	11. Chart as necessary (date, time, procedure, patient condition).
___	___	___	12. After the procedure is completed, return the room to its normal condition and replace any used equipment or supplies.

DC means done correctly.
DI means done incorrectly. (This step must be repeated and done correctly to complete the checkoff. A note is needed stating the problem and that it was corrected.)
NA means not appropriate. (This step was not needed in this procedure.)

Verbal communication with the patient: ___ satisfactory ___ unsatisfactory ___ not needed. Area(s) needing improvement:

Written communication/charting: ____satisfactory ____ unsatisfactory. Area(s) needing improvement:

_____   _____   _____   _____
Evaluator's signature   Date passed   Student's/Employee's signature   Date passed

If previous attempts were unsatisfactory, the problem(s) must be listed here with the remedial action taken to correct the problem. This must be signed by the evaluator and dated.

PROCEDURE 1 CHECKLIST
USE OF A RESUSCITATION BAG AND MASK DURING CPR

Verbal questions that must be answered correctly before starting the procedure:

1. Identify when this equipment would be needed.
2. Identify the equipment needed for adult or pediatric patients.
3. Describe why supplemental oxygen is used.
4. Identify how to clear any obstruction from the equipment.

CLINICAL checkoff on the procedure.

DC	DI	NA	
___	___	___	1. Put clean gloves on both hands; and mask and goggles as needed.
___	___	___	2. Select the proper resuscitation bag.
___	___	___	3. Select the additional equipment needed (flowmeter with tubing adapter, oxygen tubing, face mask).
___	___	___	4. Connect bag, oxygen tubing, flowmeter and face mask, if needed.
___	___	___	5. Set the proper oxygen flow on the flowmeter.
___	___	___	6. Attach bag to patient's artificial airway, if appropriate. Attach bag and face mask to patient, if appropriate.
___	___	___	7. Squeeze the bag at the appropriate rate.
___	___	___	8. Squeeze the bag to deliver an appropriate volume.
___	___	___	9. Monitor the patient's breathing, pulse, and appearance.
___	___	___	10. Report observations to proper health care personnel.
___	___	___	11. Chart as necessary (date, time, procedure, patient condition).
___	___	___	12. After the procedure is completed, return the room to its normal condition and replace any used equipment or supplies.

DC means done correctly.
DI means done incorrectly. (This step must be repeated and done correctly to complete the checkoff. A note is needed stating the problem and that it was corrected.)
NA means not appropriate. (This step was not needed in this procedure.)

Verbal communication with the patient: ___ satisfactory ___ unsatisfactory ___ not needed. Area(s) needing improvement:

Written communication/charting: ____satisfactory ____ unsatisfactory. Area(s) needing improvement:

_____   _____   _____   _____
Evaluator's signature   Date passed   Student's/Employee's signature   Date passed

If previous attempts were unsatisfactory, the problem(s) must be listed here with the remedial action taken to correct the problem. This must be signed by the evaluator and dated.

PROCEDURE 2 CHECKLIST
USE OF A MOUTH-TO-VALVE MASK (POCKET MASK) DURING CPR

Verbal questions that must be answered correctly before starting the procedure:

1. Identify when this equipment would be needed.
2. Identify the equipment needed for adult or pediatric patients.
3. Describe why supplemental oxygen is used.
4. Identify how to clear any obstruction from the equipment.

LABORATORY checkoff on the procedure.

DC	DI	NA	
___	___	___	1. Put clean gloves on both hands; and mask and goggles as needed.
___	___	___	2. Select the proper mouth-to-valve mask.
___	___	___	3. Select the additional equipment, if used (flowmeter with tubing adapter, oxygen tubing).
___	___	___	4. Assemble the valve, mask, and mouthpiece.
___	___	___	5. Connect oxygen tubing and flowmeter to mask, if used.
___	___	___	6. Set the proper oxygen flow on the flowmeter, if used.
___	___	___	7. Attach face mask to patient.
___	___	___	8. Blow into the mouthpiece at an appropriate rate.
___	___	___	9. Blow into the mouthpiece to deliver an appropriate volume.
___	___	___	10. Monitor the patient's breathing, pulse, and appearance.
___	___	___	11. Report observations to proper health care personnel.
___	___	___	12. Chart as necessary (date, time, procedure, patient condition).
___	___	___	13. After the procedure is completed, return the room to its normal condition and replace any used equipment or supplies.

DC means done correctly.
DI means done incorrectly. (This step must be repeated and done correctly to complete the checkoff. A note is needed stating the problem and that it was corrected.)
NA means not appropriate. (This step was not needed in this procedure.)

Verbal communication with the patient: ___ satisfactory ___ unsatisfactory ___ not needed.
Area(s) needing improvement:

Written communication/charting: ___ satisfactory ___ unsatisfactory. Area(s) needing improvement:

_____   _____   _____   _____
Evaluator's signature   Date passed   Student's/Employee's signature   Date passed

If previous attempts were unsatisfactory, the problem(s) must be listed here with the remedial action taken to correct the problem. This must be signed by the evaluator and dated.

PROCEDURE 2 CHECKLIST
USE OF A MOUTH-TO-VALVE MASK (POCKET MASK) DURING CPR

Verbal questions that must be answered correctly before starting the procedure:

1. Identify when this equipment would be needed.
2. Identify the equipment needed for adult or pediatric patients.
3. Describe why supplemental oxygen is used.
4. Identify how to clear any obstruction from the equipment.

CLINICAL checkoff on the procedure.

DC	DI	NA	
——	——	——	1. Put clean gloves on both hands; and mask and goggles as needed.
——	——	——	2. Select the proper mouth-to-valve mask.
——	——	——	3. Select the additional equipment, if used (flowmeter with tubing adapter, oxygen tubing).
——	——	——	4. Assemble the valve, mask, and mouthpiece.
——	——	——	5. Connect oxygen tubing and flowmeter to mask, if used.
——	——	——	6. Set the proper oxygen flow on the flowmeter, if used.
——	——	——	7. Attach face mask to patient.
——	——	——	8. Blow into the mouthpiece at an appropriate rate.
——	——	——	9. Blow into the mouthpiece to deliver an appropriate volume.
——	——	——	10. Monitor the patient's breathing, pulse, and appearance.
——	——	——	11. Report observations to proper health care personnel.
——	——	——	12. Chart as necessary (date, time, procedure, patient condition).
——	——	——	13. After the procedure is completed, return the room to its normal condition and replace any used equipment or supplies.

DC means done correctly.
DI means done incorrectly. (This step must be repeated and done correctly to complete the checkoff. A note is needed stating the problem and that it was corrected.)
NA means not appropriate. (This step was not needed in this procedure.)

Verbal communication with the patient: ___ satisfactory ___ unsatisfactory ___ not needed. Area(s) needing improvement:

Written communication/charting: ____satisfactory ____ unsatisfactory. Area(s) needing improvement:

_____   _____   _____   _____
Evaluator's signature   Date passed   Student's/Employee's signature   Date passed

If previous attempts were unsatisfactory, the problem(s) must be listed here with the remedial action taken to correct the problem. This must be signed by the evaluator and dated.

PROCEDURE 3 CHECKLIST
PULSE OXIMETRY

Verbal questions that must be answered correctly before starting the procedure:

1. What is the normal value for pulse oximetry?
2. Identify what equipment is needed.
3. Identify situations in which pulse oximetry may not give accurate results.

LABORATORY checkoff on the procedure.

DC   DI   NA

— — — 1. Confirm that the physician's order is current and complete, including a pulse oximetry goal and if the patient is to use supplemental oxygen.
— — — 2. Review the chart for current patient information.
— — — 3. Greet the patient, identify yourself, and state your purpose.
— — — 4. Confirm the patient's identity on his or her wristband.
— — — 5. Make sure the oximeter sensor is properly placed on the patient. Adjust the equipment if needed.
— — — 6. Make sure the oxygen flow or percentage is set as ordered.
— — — 7. Identify a strong signal indicating a reliable pulse oximetry reading. Get help if a reliable signal cannot be obtained.
— — — 8. Note the patient's pulse oximetry value.
— — — 9. Note the patient's pulse rate, if the instrument gives it.
— — — 10. Monitor the patient's breathing, pulse, and appearance.
— — — 11. Report observations to proper health care personnel.
— — — 12. Chart as necessary (date, time, procedure, patient condition).
— — — 13. After the procedure is completed, return the room to its normal condition and replace any used equipment or supplies.

DC means done correctly.
DI means done incorrectly. (This step must be repeated and done correctly to complete the checkoff. A note is needed stating the problem and that it was corrected.)
NA means not appropriate. (This step was not needed in this procedure.)

Verbal communication with the patient: ___ satisfactory ___ unsatisfactory ___ not needed. Area(s) needing improvement:

Written communication/charting: ____satisfactory ____ unsatisfactory. Area(s) needing improvement:

_____   _____   _____   _____
Evaluator's signature   Date passed   Student's/Employee's signature   Date passed

If previous attempts were unsatisfactory, the problem(s) must be listed here with the remedial action taken to correct the problem. This must be signed by the evaluator and dated.

PROCEDURE 3 CHECKLIST
PULSE OXIMETRY

Verbal questions that must be answered correctly before starting the procedure:

1. What is the normal value for pulse oximetry?
2. Identify what equipment is needed.
3. Identify situations in which pulse oximetry may not give accurate results.

CLINICAL checkoff on the procedure.

DC	DI	NA	
__	__	__	1. Confirm that the physician's order is current and complete, including a pulse oximetry goal and if the patient is to use supplemental oxygen.
__	__	__	2. Review the chart for current patient information.
__	__	__	3. Greet the patient, identify yourself, and state your purpose.
__	__	__	4. Confirm the patient's identity on his or her wristband.
__	__	__	5. Make sure the oximeter sensor is properly placed on the patient. Adjust the equipment if needed.
__	__	__	6. Make sure the oxygen flow or percentage is set as ordered.
__	__	__	7. Identify a strong signal indicating a reliable pulse oximetry reading. Get help if a reliable signal cannot be obtained.
__	__	__	8. Note the patient's pulse oximetry value.
__	__	__	9. Note the patient's pulse rate, if the instrument gives it.
__	__	__	10. Monitor the patient's breathing, pulse, and appearance.
__	__	__	11. Report observations to proper health care personnel.
__	__	__	12. Chart as necessary (date, time, procedure, patient condition).
__	__	__	13. After the procedure is completed, return the room to its normal condition and replace any used equipment or supplies.

DC means done correctly.
DI means done incorrectly. (This step must be repeated and done correctly to complete the checkoff. A note is needed stating the problem and that it was corrected.)
NA means not appropriate. (This step was not needed in this procedure.)

Verbal communication with the patient: ___ satisfactory ___ unsatisfactory ___ not needed. Area(s) needing improvement:

Written communication/charting: ____satisfactory ____ unsatisfactory. Area(s) needing improvement:

_____   _____   _____   _____
Evaluator's signature   Date passed   Student's/Employee's signature   Date passed

If previous attempts were unsatisfactory, the problem(s) must be listed here with the remedial action taken to correct the problem. This must be signed by the evaluator and dated.

PROCEDURE 4 CHECKLIST
MAINTENANCE OF A NASAL CANNULA

Verbal questions that must be answered correctly before starting the procedure:

1. Give at least one reason why supplemental oxygen would be ordered.
2. Identify safety rules when oxygen is being used.

LABORATORY checkoff on the procedure.

DC	DI	NA	
___	___	___	1. Confirm that the physician's order is current and complete.
___	___	___	2. Review the chart for current patient information.
___	___	___	3. Greet the patient, identify yourself, and state your purpose.
___	___	___	4. Confirm the patient's identity on his or her wristband.
___	___	___	5. Wash your hands.
___	___	___	6. Make sure the equipment is properly placed on the patient. Adjust the equipment if needed.
___	___	___	7. Make sure the oxygen flowmeter is set as ordered. If not, get your supervisor or the RN or RCP.
___	___	___	8. If a humidifier is in use, check for adequate water in the bottle.
___	___	___	9. If a humidifier is in use, check that the pressure relief valve is operating normally.
___	___	___	10. Reinforce to the patient the need to keep the nasal cannula in place at all times and to observe the oxygen safety rules.
___	___	___	11. Monitor the patient's breathing, pulse, and appearance.
___	___	___	12. Report observations to proper health care personnel.
___	___	___	13. Chart as necessary (date, time, procedure, patient condition).
___	___	___	14. After the procedure is completed, return the room to its normal condition and replace any used equipment or supplies.

DC means done correctly.
DI means done incorrectly. (This step must be repeated and done correctly to complete the checkoff. A note is needed stating the problem and that it was corrected.)
NA means not appropriate. (This step was not needed in this procedure.)

Verbal communication with the patient: ___ satisfactory ___ unsatisfactory ___ not needed. Area(s) needing improvement:

Written communication/charting: ____satisfactory ____ unsatisfactory. Area(s) needing improvement:

_____   _____   _____   _____
Evaluator's signature   Date passed   Student's/Employee's signature   Date passed

If previous attempts were unsatisfactory, the problem(s) must be listed here with the remedial action taken to correct the problem. This must be signed by the evaluator and dated.

PROCEDURE 4 CHECKLIST
MAINTENANCE OF A NASAL CANNULA

Verbal questions that must be answered correctly before starting the procedure:

1. Give at least one reason why supplemental oxygen would be ordered.
2. Identify safety rules when oxygen is being used.

CLINICAL checkoff on the procedure.

DC	DI	NA	
___	___	___	1. Confirm that the physician's order is current and complete.
___	___	___	2. Review the chart for current patient information.
___	___	___	3. Greet the patient, identify yourself, and state your purpose.
___	___	___	4. Confirm the patient's identity on his or her wristband.
___	___	___	5. Wash your hands.
___	___	___	6. Make sure the equipment is properly placed on the patient. Adjust the equipment if needed.
___	___	___	7. Make sure the oxygen flowmeter is set as ordered. If not, get your supervisor or the RN or RCP.
___	___	___	8. If a humidifier is in use, check for adequate water in the bottle.
___	___	___	9. If a humidifier is in use, check that the pressure relief valve is operating normally.
___	___	___	10. Reinforce to the patient the need to keep the nasal cannula in place at all times and to observe the oxygen safety rules.
___	___	___	11. Monitor the patient's breathing, pulse, and appearance.
___	___	___	12. Report observations to proper health care personnel.
___	___	___	13. Chart as necessary (date, time, procedure, patient condition).
___	___	___	14. After the procedure is completed, return the room to its normal condition and replace any used equipment or supplies.

DC means done correctly.
DI means done incorrectly. (This step must be repeated and done correctly to complete the checkoff. A note is needed stating the problem and that it was corrected.)
NA means not appropriate. (This step was not needed in this procedure.)

Verbal communication with the patient: ___ satisfactory ___ unsatisfactory ___ not needed. Area(s) needing improvement:

Written communication/charting: ___satisfactory ___ unsatisfactory. Area(s) needing improvement:

_____   _____   _____   _____
Evaluator's signature   Date passed   Student's/Employee's signature   Date passed

If previous attempts were unsatisfactory, the problem(s) must be listed here with the remedial action taken to correct the problem. This must be signed by the evaluator and dated.

PROCEDURE 5 CHECKLIST
MAINTENANCE OF AN AIR ENTRAINMENT (VENTURI) MASK

Verbal questions that must be answered correctly before starting the procedure:

1. Give at least one reason why supplemental oxygen would be ordered.
2. Identify safety rules when oxygen is being used.
3. Identify special considerations for the proper use of this type of oxygen mask.

LABORATORY checkoff on the procedure.

DC	DI	NA	
___	___	___	1. Confirm that the physician's order is current and complete.
___	___	___	2. Review the chart for current patient information.
___	___	___	3. Greet the patient, identify yourself, and state your purpose.
___	___	___	4. Confirm the patient's identity on his or her wristband.
___	___	___	5. Wash your hands.
___	___	___	6. Make sure the equipment is properly placed on the patient. Adjust the equipment if needed.
___	___	___	7. Make sure the oxygen flowmeter is turned on and set as ordered. If not, get your supervisor or the RN or RCP.
___	___	___	8. If a humidifier is in use, check for adequate water in the bottle.
___	___	___	9. If a humidifier is in use, check that the pressure relief valve is operating normally.
___	___	___	10. Reinforce to the patient the need to keep the mask in place at all times, to not adjust it or cover it up, and to observe the oxygen safety rules.
___	___	___	11. Monitor the patient's breathing, pulse, and appearance.
___	___	___	12. Report observations to proper health care personnel.
___	___	___	13. Chart as necessary (date, time, procedure, patient condition).
___	___	___	14. After the procedure is completed, return the room to its normal condition and replace any used equipment or supplies.

DC means done correctly.
DI means done incorrectly. (This step must be repeated and done correctly to complete the checkoff. A note is needed stating the problem and that it was corrected.)
NA means not appropriate. (This step was not needed in this procedure.)

Verbal communication with the patient: ___ satisfactory ___ unsatisfactory ___ not needed. Area(s) needing improvement:

Written communication/charting: ____satisfactory ____ unsatisfactory. Area(s) needing improvement:

_____   _____   _____   _____
Evaluator's signature   Date passed   Student's/Employee's signature   Date passed

If previous attempts were unsatisfactory, the problem(s) must be listed here with the remedial action taken to correct the problem. This must be signed by the evaluator and dated.

PROCEDURE 5 CHECKLIST
MAINTENANCE OF AN AIR ENTRAINMENT (VENTURI) MASK

Verbal questions that must be answered correctly before starting the procedure:

1. Give at least one reason why supplemental oxygen would be ordered.
2. Identify safety rules when oxygen is being used.
3. Identify special considerations for the proper use of this type of oxygen mask.

CLINICAL checkoff on the procedure.

DC   DI   NA

___ ___ ___   1. Confirm that the physician's order is current and complete.
___ ___ ___   2. Review the chart for current patient information.
___ ___ ___   3. Greet the patient, identify yourself, and state your purpose.
___ ___ ___   4. Confirm the patient's identity on his or her wristband.
___ ___ ___   5. Wash your hands.
___ ___ ___   6. Make sure the equipment is properly placed on the patient. Adjust the equipment if needed.
___ ___ ___   7. Make sure the oxygen flowmeter is turned on and set as ordered. If not, get your supervisor or the RN or RCP.
___ ___ ___   8. If a humidifier is in use, check for adequate water in the bottle.
___ ___ ___   9. If a humidifier is in use, check that the pressure relief valve is operating normally.
___ ___ ___ 10. Reinforce to the patient the need to keep the mask in place at all times, to not adjust it or cover it up, and to observe the oxygen safety rules.
___ ___ ___ 11. Monitor the patient's breathing, pulse, and appearance.
___ ___ ___ 12. Report observations to proper health care personnel.
___ ___ ___ 13. Chart as necessary (date, time, procedure, patient condition).
___ ___ ___ 14. After the procedure is completed, return the room to its normal condition and replace any used equipment or supplies.

DC means done correctly.
DI means done incorrectly. (This step must be repeated and done correctly to complete the checkoff. A note is needed stating the problem and that it was corrected.)
NA means not appropriate. (This step was not needed in this procedure.)

Verbal communication with the patient: ___ satisfactory ___ unsatisfactory ___ not needed. Area(s) needing improvement:

Written communication/charting: ____satisfactory ____ unsatisfactory. Area(s) needing improvement:

_____   _____   _____   _____
Evaluator's signature   Date passed   Student's/Employee's signature   Date passed

If previous attempts were unsatisfactory, the problem(s) must be listed here with the remedial action taken to correct the problem. This must be signed by the evaluator and dated.

PROCEDURE 6 CHECKLIST
MAINTENANCE OF A SIMPLE OXYGEN MASK

Verbal questions that must be answered correctly before starting the procedure:

1. Give at least one reason why supplemental oxygen would be ordered.
2. Identify safety rules when oxygen is being used.
3. Identify special considerations for the proper use of this type of oxygen mask.

LABORATORY checkoff on the procedure.

DC	DI	NA	
___	___	___	1. Confirm that the physician's order is current and complete.
___	___	___	2. Review the chart for current patient information.
___	___	___	3. Greet the patient, identify yourself, and state your purpose.
___	___	___	4. Confirm the patient's identity on his or her wristband.
___	___	___	5. Wash your hands.
___	___	___	6. Make sure the equipment is properly placed on the patient. Adjust the equipment if needed.
___	___	___	7. Make sure the oxygen flowmeter is set as ordered and turned on. If not, get your supervisor or the RN or RCP.
___	___	___	8. If a humidifier is in use, add sterile water to it as indicated.
___	___	___	9. If a humidifier is in use, check that the pressure relief valve is operating normally.
___	___	___	10. Reinforce to the patient the need to keep the oxygen mask in place at all times, to not cover it up, and to observe the oxygen safety rules.
___	___	___	11. Monitor the patient's breathing, pulse, and appearance.
___	___	___	12. Report observations to proper health care personnel.
___	___	___	13. Chart as necessary (date, time, procedure, patient condition).
___	___	___	14. After the procedure is completed, return the room to its normal condition and replace any used equipment or supplies.

DC means done correctly.
DI means done incorrectly. (This step must be repeated and done correctly to complete the checkoff. A note is needed stating the problem and that it was corrected.)
NA means not appropriate. (This step was not needed in this procedure.)

Verbal communication with the patient: ___ satisfactory ___ unsatisfactory ___ not needed.
Area(s) needing improvement:

Written communication/charting: ____satisfactory ____ unsatisfactory. Area(s) needing improvement:

_____   _____   _____   _____
Evaluator's signature   Date passed   Student's/Employee's signature   Date passed

If previous attempts were unsatisfactory, the problem(s) must be listed here with the remedial action taken to correct the problem. This must be signed by the evaluator and dated.

PROCEDURE 6 CHECKLIST
MAINTENANCE OF A SIMPLE OXYGEN MASK

Verbal questions that must be answered correctly before starting the procedure:

1. Give at least one reason why supplemental oxygen would be ordered.
2. Identify safety rules when oxygen is being used.
3. Identify special considerations for the proper use of this type of oxygen mask.

CLINICAL checkoff on the procedure.

DC	DI	NA	
___	___	___	1. Confirm that the physician's order is current and complete.
___	___	___	2. Review the chart for current patient information.
___	___	___	3. Greet the patient, identify yourself, and state your purpose.
___	___	___	4. Confirm the patient's identity on his or her wristband.
___	___	___	5. Wash your hands.
___	___	___	6. Make sure the equipment is properly placed on the patient. Adjust the equipment if needed.
___	___	___	7. Make sure the oxygen flowmeter is set as ordered and turned on. If not, get your supervisor or the RN or RCP.
___	___	___	8. If a humidifier is in use, add sterile water to it as indicated.
___	___	___	9. If a humidifier is in use, check that the pressure relief valve is operating normally.
___	___	___	10. Reinforce to the patient the need to keep the oxygen mask in place at all times, to not cover it up, and to observe the oxygen safety rules.
___	___	___	11. Monitor the patient's breathing, pulse, and appearance.
___	___	___	12. Report observations to proper health care personnel.
___	___	___	13. Chart as necessary (date, time, procedure, patient condition).
___	___	___	14. After the procedure is completed, return the room to its normal condition and replace any used equipment or supplies.

DC means done correctly.
DI means done incorrectly. (This step must be repeated and done correctly to complete the checkoff. A note is needed stating the problem and that it was corrected.)
NA means not appropriate. (This step was not needed in this procedure.)

Verbal communication with the patient: ___ satisfactory ___ unsatisfactory ___ not needed. Area(s) needing improvement:

Written communication/charting: ____satisfactory ____ unsatisfactory. Area(s) needing improvement:

_____   _____   _____   _____
Evaluator's signature   Date passed   Student's/Employee's signature   Date passed

If previous attempts were unsatisfactory, the problem(s) must be listed here with the remedial action taken to correct the problem. This must be signed by the evaluator and dated.

PROCEDURE 7 CHECKLIST
MAINTENANCE OF A NONREBREATHER MASK

Verbal questions that must be answered correctly before starting the procedure:

1. Give at least one reason why supplemental oxygen would be ordered.
2. Identify safety rules when oxygen is being used.
3. Identify special considerations for the proper use of this type of oxygen mask.

LABORATORY checkoff on the procedure.

DC	DI	NA	
——	——	——	1. Confirm that the physician's order is current and complete.
——	——	——	2. Review the chart for current patient information.
——	——	——	3. Greet the patient, identify yourself, and state your purpose.
——	——	——	4. Confirm the patient's identity on his or her wristband.
——	——	——	5. Wash your hands.
——	——	——	6. Make sure the equipment is properly placed on the patient. Adjust the equipment if needed.
——	——	——	7. Make sure the reservoir bag does not collapse by more than one-half during inspiration. Get the RCP if the bag collapses by more than one-half.
——	——	——	8. If a humidifier is in use, check for adequate water in the bottle.
——	——	——	9. If a humidifier is in use, check that the pressure relief valve is operating normally.
——	——	——	10. Reinforce to the patient the need to keep the mask in place at all times, to not cover it up, and to observe the oxygen safety rules.
——	——	——	11. Monitor the patient's breathing, pulse, and appearance.
——	——	——	12. Report observations to proper health care personnel.
——	——	——	13. Chart as necessary (date, time, procedure, patient condition).
——	——	——	14. After the procedure is completed, return the room to its normal condition and replace any used equipment or supplies.

DC means done correctly.
DI means done incorrectly. (This step must be repeated and done correctly to complete the checkoff. A note is needed stating the problem and that it was corrected.)
NA means not appropriate. (This step was not needed in this procedure.)

Verbal communication with the patient: ___ satisfactory ___ unsatisfactory ___ not needed. Area(s) needing improvement:

Written communication/charting: ____satisfactory ____ unsatisfactory. Area(s) needing improvement:

_____   _____   _____   _____
Evaluator's signature   Date passed   Student's/Employee's signature   Date passed

If previous attempts were unsatisfactory, the problem(s) must be listed here with the remedial action taken to correct the problem. This must be signed by the evaluator and dated.

PROCEDURE 7 CHECKLIST
MAINTENANCE OF A NONREBREATHER MASK

Verbal questions that must be answered correctly before starting the procedure:

1. Give at least one reason why supplemental oxygen would be ordered.
2. Identify safety rules when oxygen is being used.
3. Identify special considerations for the proper use of this type of oxygen mask.

CLINICAL checkoff on the procedure.

DC	DI	NA	
——	——	——	1. Confirm that the physician's order is current and complete.
——	——	——	2. Review the chart for current patient information.
——	——	——	3. Greet the patient, identify yourself, and state your purpose.
——	——	——	4. Confirm the patient's identity on his or her wristband.
——	——	——	5. Wash your hands.
——	——	——	6. Make sure the equipment is properly placed on the patient. Adjust the equipment if needed.
——	——	——	7. Make sure the reservoir bag does not collapse by more than one-half during inspiration. Get the RCP if the bag collapses by more than one-half.
——	——	——	8. If a humidifier is in use, check for adequate water in the bottle.
——	——	——	9. If a humidifier is in use, check that the pressure relief valve is operating normally.
——	——	——	10. Reinforce to the patient the need to keep the mask in place at all times, to not cover it up, and to observe the oxygen safety rules.
——	——	——	11. Monitor the patient's breathing, pulse, and appearance.
——	——	——	12. Report observations to proper health care personnel.
——	——	——	13. Chart as necessary (date, time, procedure, patient condition).
——	——	——	14. After the procedure is completed, return the room to its normal condition and replace any used equipment or supplies.

DC means done correctly.
DI means done incorrectly. (This step must be repeated and done correctly to complete the checkoff. A note is needed stating the problem and that it was corrected.)
NA means not appropriate. (This step was not needed in this procedure.)

Verbal communication with the patient: ___ satisfactory ___ unsatisfactory ___ not needed. Area(s) needing improvement:

Written communication/charting: ____satisfactory ____ unsatisfactory. Area(s) needing improvement:

_____   _____   _____   _____
Evaluator's signature   Date passed   Student's/Employee's signature   Date passed

If previous attempts were unsatisfactory, the problem(s) must be listed here with the remedial action taken to correct the problem. This must be signed by the evaluator and dated.

PROCEDURE 8 CHECKLIST
INCENTIVE SPIROMETRY

Verbal questions that must be answered correctly before starting the procedure:

1. Identify why patients receive this therapy.
2. Describe how the patient should breathe during incentive spirometry.
3. Identify complications that may occur during an incentive spirometry treatment.

LABORATORY checkoff on the procedure.

DC	DI	NA	
___	___	___	1. Confirm that the physician's order is current and complete.
___	___	___	2. Review the chart for current patient information.
___	___	___	3. Greet the patient, identify yourself, and state your purpose.
___	___	___	4. Confirm the patient's identity on his or her wristband.
___	___	___	5. Wash your hands.
___	___	___	6. Make sure the equipment is properly set up for the patient. Adjust the equipment if needed.
___	___	___	7. If a target volume or target flow has been chosen, set it for the patient.
___	___	___	8. Ask the patient to exhale normally and then inhale as deeply as possible and hold the breath for 3 to 4 seconds.
___	___	___	9. Note the patient's inhaled volume and breath hold time.
___	___	___	10. Encourage the patient to cough deeply.
___	___	___	11. Encourage the patient to perform a proper incentive spirometry breath the number of times per hour that the physician has ordered.
___	___	___	12. Monitor the patient's breathing, pulse, and appearance.
___	___	___	13. Report observations to proper health care personnel.
___	___	___	14. Chart as necessary (date, time, procedure, patient condition).
___	___	___	15. After the procedure is completed, return the room to its normal condition and replace any used equipment or supplies.

DC means done correctly.
DI means done incorrectly. (This step must be repeated and done correctly to complete the checkoff. A note is needed stating the problem and that it was corrected.)
NA means not appropriate. (This step was not needed in this procedure.)

Verbal communication with the patient: ___ satisfactory ___ unsatisfactory ___ not needed. Area(s) needing improvement:

Written communication/charting: ____satisfactory ____ unsatisfactory. Area(s) needing improvement:

_____   _____   _____   _____
Evaluator's signature   Date passed   Student's/Employee's signature   Date passed

If previous attempts were unsatisfactory, the problem(s) must be listed here with the remedial action taken to correct the problem. This must be signed by the evaluator and dated.

PROCEDURE 8 CHECKLIST
INCENTIVE SPIROMETRY

Verbal questions that must be answered correctly before starting the procedure:

1. Identify why patients receive this therapy.
2. Describe how the patient should breathe during incentive spirometry.
3. Identify complications that may occur during an incentive spirometry treatment.

CLINICAL checkoff on the procedure.

DC	DI	NA	
__	__	__	1. Confirm that the physician's order is current and complete.
__	__	__	2. Review the chart for current patient information.
__	__	__	3. Greet the patient, identify yourself, and state your purpose.
__	__	__	4. Confirm the patient's identity on his or her wristband.
__	__	__	5. Wash your hands.
__	__	__	6. Make sure the equipment is properly set up for the patient. Adjust the equipment if needed.
__	__	__	7. If a target volume or target flow has been chosen, set it for the patient.
__	__	__	8. Ask the patient to exhale normally and then inhale as deeply as possible and hold the breath for 3 to 4 seconds.
__	__	__	9. Note the patient's inhaled volume and breath hold time.
__	__	__	10. Encourage the patient to cough deeply.
__	__	__	11. Encourage the patient to perform a proper incentive spirometry breath the number of times per hour that the physician has ordered.
__	__	__	12. Monitor the patient's breathing, pulse, and appearance.
__	__	__	13. Report observations to proper health care personnel.
__	__	__	14. Chart as necessary (date, time, procedure, patient condition).
__	__	__	15. After the procedure is completed, return the room to its normal condition and replace any used equipment or supplies.

DC means done correctly.
DI means done incorrectly. (This step must be repeated and done correctly to complete the checkoff. A note is needed stating the problem and that it was corrected.)
NA means not appropriate. (This step was not needed in this procedure.)

Verbal communication with the patient: ___ satisfactory ___ unsatisfactory ___ not needed.
Area(s) needing improvement:

Written communication/charting: ____satisfactory ____ unsatisfactory. Area(s) needing improvement:

_____   _____   _____   _____
Evaluator's signature   Date passed   Student's/Employee's signature   Date passed

If previous attempts were unsatisfactory, the problem(s) must be listed here with the remedial action taken to correct the problem. This must be signed by the evaluator and dated.

PROCEDURE 9 CHECKLIST
COUGH AND DEEP BREATHING EXERCISES

Verbal questions that must be answered correctly before starting the procedure:

1. Identify why patients receive this therapy.
2. Describe how the patient should breathe during this exercise.
3. Identify a consequence of performing this exercise with a recent postoperative patient.

LABORATORY checkoff on the procedure.

DC	DI	NA	
___	___	___	1. Confirm that the physician's order is current and complete.
___	___	___	2. Review the chart for current patient information.
___	___	___	3. Greet the patient, identify yourself, and state your purpose.
___	___	___	4. Confirm the patient's identity on his or her wristband.
___	___	___	5. Wash your hands.
___	___	___	6. Get a pillow or blanket to support an incision, if needed.
___	___	___	7. Position a bedbound patient with head elevated for comfort, bent knees, and hands or pillow supporting a chest or abdominal incision.
___	___	___	8. Have the patient breathe two or three times in through the nose and out through the mouth.
___	___	___	9. Have the patient inhale as much as possible and perform as strong a cough as possible.
___	___	___	10. Have the patient cough out any sputum that is produced.
___	___	___	11. Note the amount, color, odor, and consistency of the sputum.
___	___	___	12. Monitor the patient's breathing, pulse, and appearance.
___	___	___	13. Report observations to proper health care personnel.
___	___	___	14. Chart as necessary (date, time, procedure, patient condition).
___	___	___	15. After the procedure is completed, return the patient to his or her former position and the room to its normal condition.

DC means done correctly.
DI means done incorrectly. (This step must be repeated and done correctly to complete the checkoff. A note is needed stating the problem and that it was corrected.)
NA means not appropriate. (This step was not needed in this procedure.)

Verbal communication with the patient: ___ satisfactory ___ unsatisfactory ___ not needed. Area(s) needing improvement:

Written communication/charting: ____satisfactory ____ unsatisfactory. Area(s) needing improvement:

_____   _____   _____   _____
Evaluator's signature   Date passed   Student's/Employee's signature   Date passed

If previous attempts were unsatisfactory, the problem(s) must be listed here with the remedial action taken to correct the problem. This must be signed by the evaluator and dated.

PROCEDURE 9 CHECKLIST
COUGH AND DEEP BREATHING EXERCISES

Verbal questions that must be answered correctly before starting the procedure:

1. Identify why patients receive this therapy.
2. Describe how the patient should breathe during this exercise.
3. Identify a consequence of performing this exercise with a recent postoperative patient.

CLINICAL checkoff on the procedure.

DC	DI	NA	
___	___	___	1. Confirm that the physician's order is current and complete.
___	___	___	2. Review the chart for current patient information.
___	___	___	3. Greet the patient, identify yourself, and state your purpose.
___	___	___	4. Confirm the patient's identity on his or her wristband.
___	___	___	5. Wash your hands.
___	___	___	6. Get a pillow or blanket to support an incision, if needed.
___	___	___	7. Position a bedbound patient with head elevated for comfort, bent knees, and hands or pillow supporting a chest or abdominal incision.
___	___	___	8. Have the patient breathe two or three times in through the nose and out through the mouth.
___	___	___	9. Have the patient inhale as much as possible and perform as strong a cough as possible.
___	___	___	10. Have the patient cough out any sputum that is produced.
___	___	___	11. Note the amount, color, odor, and consistency of the sputum.
___	___	___	12. Monitor the patient's breathing, pulse, and appearance.
___	___	___	13. Report observations to proper health care personnel.
___	___	___	14. Chart as necessary (date, time, procedure, patient condition).
___	___	___	15. After the procedure is completed, return the patient to his or her former position and the room to its normal condition.

DC means done correctly.
DI means done incorrectly. (This step must be repeated and done correctly to complete the checkoff. A note is needed stating the problem and that it was corrected.)
NA means not appropriate. (This step was not needed in this procedure.)

Verbal communication with the patient: ___ satisfactory ___ unsatisfactory ___ not needed. Area(s) needing improvement:

Written communication/charting: ____ satisfactory ____ unsatisfactory. Area(s) needing improvement:

_____   _____   _____   _____
Evaluator's signature   Date passed   Student's/Employee's signature   Date passed

If previous attempts were unsatisfactory, the problem(s) must be listed here with the remedial action taken to correct the problem. This must be signed by the evaluator and dated.

PROCEDURE 10 CHECKLIST
CHANGING A PORTABLE "E" TYPE TANK OF OXYGEN

Verbal questions that must be answered correctly before starting the procedure:

1. Describe how to determine that the contents of a tank are oxygen.
2. Identify the safety precautions to be used with tanks of oxygen.
3. Identify the pressure that indicates an oxygen tank should be replaced.

LABORATORY checkoff on the procedure.

DC	DI	NA	
___	___	___	1. Slowly turn on the old tank to check its pressure and confirm that it is empty. (It is acceptable to turn on the tank and state the pressure at which a tank should be changed.)
___	___	___	2. Turn off the tank.
___	___	___	3. Turn on the flowmeter to bleed the pressure out of the regulator.
___	___	___	4. Turn off the flowmeter.
___	___	___	5. Remove the regulator from the tank.
___	___	___	6. Remove and discard the old plastic washer from the regulator.
___	___	___	7. Label the tank as EMPTY. Store it securely.
___	___	___	8. Select a replacement tank by confirming that the adhesive label states that it contains oxygen and that the tank is painted green in color.
___	___	___	9. Remove the plastic protective covering from the new tank.
___	___	___	10. Place the new plastic washer from the protective covering on the regulator.
___	___	___	11. **Slowly** turn on the tank to crack it and blow any dust from the oxygen outlet. Turn off the tank.
___	___	___	12. Place and tighten the regulator onto the new tank.
___	___	___	13. Slowly turn on the tank and make sure there is no leak around the regulator. Tighten the regulator if needed.
___	___	___	14. Note the pressure in the tank to confirm that it is full (about 2,000 psi).
___	___	___	15. Turn off the tank by turning the tank wrench counterclockwise.
___	___	___	16. Turn on the flowmeter to bleed the pressure from the regulator.
___	___	___	17. Turn off the flowmeter.
___	___	___	18. Put the tank in a secure place (tank cart, tank rack on wheelchair or transport gurney, or chained to wall).

DC means done correctly.
DI means done incorrectly. (This step must be repeated and done correctly to complete the checkoff. A note is needed stating the problem and that it was corrected.)
NA means not appropriate. (This step was not needed in this procedure.)

Verbal communication with the patient: ___ satisfactory ___ unsatisfactory ___ not needed. Area(s) needing improvement:

Written communication/charting: ___satisfactory ___ unsatisfactory. Area(s) needing improvement:

_____   _____   _____   _____
Evaluator's signature   Date passed   Student's/Employee's signature   Date passed

If previous attempts were unsatisfactory, the problem(s) must be listed here with the remedial action taken to correct the problem. This must be signed by the evaluator and dated.

PROCEDURE 10 CHECKLIST
CHANGING A PORTABLE "E" TYPE TANK OF OXYGEN

Verbal questions that must be answered correctly before starting the procedure:

1. Describe how to determine that the contents of a tank are oxygen.
2. Identify the safety precautions to be used with tanks of oxygen.
3. Identify the pressure that indicates an oxygen tank should be replaced.

CLINICAL checkoff on the procedure.

DC	DI	NA	
___	___	___	1. Slowly turn on the old tank to check its pressure and confirm that it is empty. (It is acceptable to turn on the tank and state the pressure at which a tank should be changed.)
___	___	___	2. Turn off the tank.
___	___	___	3. Turn on the flowmeter to bleed the pressure out of the regulator.
___	___	___	4. Turn off the flowmeter.
___	___	___	5. Remove the regulator from the tank.
___	___	___	6. Remove and discard the old plastic washer from the regulator.
___	___	___	7. Label the tank as EMPTY. Store it securely.
___	___	___	8. Select a replacement tank by confirming that the adhesive label states that it contains oxygen and that the tank is painted green in color.
___	___	___	9. Remove the plastic protective covering from the new tank.
___	___	___	10. Place the new plastic washer from the protective covering on the regulator.
___	___	___	11. **Slowly** turn on the tank to crack it and blow any dust from the oxygen outlet. Turn off the tank.
___	___	___	12. Place and tighten the regulator onto the new tank.
___	___	___	13. Slowly turn on the tank and make sure there is no leak around the regulator. Tighten the regulator if needed.
___	___	___	14. Note the pressure in the tank to confirm that it is full (about 2,000 psi).
___	___	___	15. Turn off the tank by turning the tank wrench counterclockwise.
___	___	___	16. Turn on the flowmeter to bleed the pressure from the regulator.
___	___	___	17. Turn off the flowmeter.
___	___	___	18. Put the tank in a secure place (tank cart, tank rack on wheelchair or transport gurney, or chained to wall).

DC means done correctly.
DI means done incorrectly. (This step must be repeated and done correctly to complete the checkoff. A note is needed stating the problem and that it was corrected.)
NA means not appropriate. (This step was not needed in this procedure.)

Verbal communication with the patient: ___ satisfactory ___ unsatisfactory ___ not needed. Area(s) needing improvement:

Written communication/charting: ____satisfactory ____ unsatisfactory. Area(s) needing improvement:

_____   _____   _____   _____
Evaluator's signature   Date passed   Student's/Employee's signature   Date passed

If previous attempts were unsatisfactory, the problem(s) must be listed here with the remedial action taken to correct the problem. This must be signed by the evaluator and dated.

PROCEDURE 11 CHECKLIST
PREPARING A PORTABLE "E" TYPE TANK OF OXYGEN FOR PATIENT TRANSPORT

Note: *This procedure should not be attempted until Procedure 10 has been completed.*

Verbal questions that must be answered correctly before starting the procedure:

1. Describe how to determine that the contents of a tank are oxygen.
2. Identify the safety precautions to be used with tanks of oxygen.
3. Identify any extra equipment that may be needed for the transportation.

LABORATORY checkoff on the procedure.

DC   DI   NA

___ ___ ___   1. Confirm that the patient will need a portable oxygen tank for
        transportation.

___ ___ ___   2. Greet the patient, identify yourself, and state your purpose.

___ ___ ___   3. Confirm the patient's identity on his or her wristband.

___ ___ ___   4. Find out the type of oxygen delivery system the patient is using.

___ ___ ___   5. Find out the oxygen flow that will be needed.

___ ___ ___   6. Find out if a humidifier is being used with the oxygen delivery
        system.

___ ___ ___   7. Slowly turn on the tank to make sure it is full enough for the
        transport. (It must have at least 500 psi.)

___ ___ ___   8. If a humidifier is needed, unscrew it (with the oxygen delivery
        system) from the patient's room oxygen flowmeter and screw
        it onto the flowmeter on the oxygen tank.

___ ___ ___   9. If no humidifier is needed, unscrew the oxygen tubing adapter
        (with the oxygen delivery system) from the room oxygen
        flowmeter and screw the oxygen tubing adapter onto the
        flowmeter on the oxygen tank.

___ ___ ___   10. Turn on the tank's flowmeter to the needed oxygen flow. Turn
        off the room oxygen flowmeter.

___ ___ ___   11. Make sure the patient's oxygen delivery system is operating
        normally.

___ ___ ___   12. Keep the oxygen tank in a vertical position if a humidifier is
        used.

___ ___ ___   13. Monitor the patient's breathing, pulse, and appearance.

___ ___ ___   14. Report observations to proper health care personnel.

___ ___ ___   15. Chart as necessary (date, time, procedure, patient condition).

___ ___ ___   16. After the procedure is completed, return the patient to his or her
        former position and the room to its normal condition.

DC means done correctly.
DI means done incorrectly. (This step must be repeated and done correctly to complete the
    checkoff. A note is needed stating the problem and that it was corrected.)
NA means not appropriate. (This step was not needed in this procedure.)

Verbal communication with the patient: ___ satisfactory ___ unsatisfactory ___ not needed.
Area(s) needing improvement:

Written communication/charting: ____satisfactory ____ unsatisfactory. Area(s) needing
improvement:

_____   _____   _____   _____
Evaluator's signature   Date passed   Student's/Employee's signature   Date passed

If previous attempts were unsatisfactory, the problem(s) must be listed here with the remedial
action taken to correct the problem. This must be signed by the evaluator and dated.

PROCEDURE 11 CHECKLIST
PREPARING A PORTABLE "E" TYPE TANK OF OXYGEN FOR PATIENT TRANSPORT

Note: *This procedure should not be attempted until Procedure 10 has been completed.*

Verbal questions that must be answered correctly before starting the procedure:

1. Describe how to determine that the contents of a tank are oxygen.
2. Identify the safety precautions to be used with tanks of oxygen.
3. Identify any extra equipment that may be needed for the transportation.

CLINICAL checkoff on the procedure.

DC   DI   NA

___ ___ ___   1. Confirm that the patient will need a portable oxygen tank for
transportation.

___ ___ ___   2. Greet the patient, identify yourself, and state your purpose.

___ ___ ___   3. Confirm the patient's identity on his or her wristband.

___ ___ ___   4. Find out the type of oxygen delivery system the patient is using.

___ ___ ___   5. Find out the oxygen flow that will be needed.

___ ___ ___   6. Find out if a humidifier is being used with the oxygen delivery
system.

___ ___ ___   7. Slowly turn on the tank to make sure it is full enough for the
transport. (It must have at least 500 psi.)

___ ___ ___   8. If a humidifier is needed, unscrew it (with the oxygen delivery
system) from the patient's room oxygen flowmeter and screw
it onto the flowmeter on the oxygen tank.

___ ___ ___   9. If no humidifier is needed, unscrew the oxygen tubing adapter
(with the oxygen delivery system) from the room oxygen
flowmeter and screw the oxygen tubing adapter onto the
flowmeter on the oxygen tank.

___ ___ ___ 10. Turn on the tank's flowmeter to the needed oxygen flow. Turn
off the room oxygen flowmeter.

___ ___ ___ 11. Make sure the patient's oxygen delivery system is operating
normally.

___ ___ ___ 12. Keep the oxygen tank in a vertical position if a humidifier is
used.

___ ___ ___ 13. Monitor the patient's breathing, pulse, and appearance.

___ ___ ___ 14. Report observations to proper health care personnel.

___ ___ ___ 15. Chart as necessary (date, time, procedure, patient condition).

___ ___ ___ 16. After the procedure is completed, return the patient to his or her
former position and the room to its normal condition.

DC means done correctly.
DI means done incorrectly. (This step must be repeated and done correctly to complete the
checkoff. A note is needed stating the problem and that it was corrected.)
NA means not appropriate. (This step was not needed in this procedure.)

Verbal communication with the patient: ___ satisfactory ___ unsatisfactory ___ not needed.
Area(s) needing improvement:

Written communication/charting: ____satisfactory ____ unsatisfactory. Area(s) needing
improvement:

_____   _____   _____   _____
Evaluator's signature   Date passed   Student's/Employee's signature   Date passed

If previous attempts were unsatisfactory, the problem(s) must be listed here with the remedial
action taken to correct the problem. This must be signed by the evaluator and dated.

PROCEDURE 12 CHECKLIST
OROPHARYNGEAL SUCTIONING

Verbal questions that must be answered correctly before starting the procedure:

1. Identify the possible complication of oropharyngeal suctioning.
2. Identify the equipment needed for oropharyngeal suctioning.
3. What two things could cause a loss of vacuum?
4. What would you do if a patient needed deep tracheal suctioning?

LABORATORY checkoff on the procedure.

DC	DI	NA	
—	—	—	1. Confirm that the physician's order is current and complete.
—	—	—	2. Review the chart for current patient information.
—	—	—	3. Greet the patient, identify yourself, and state your purpose.
—	—	—	4. Confirm the patient's identity on his or her wristband.
—	—	—	5. Wash your hands and put on clean gloves, goggles, and mask according to your unit's policy.
—	—	—	6. Gather and assemble the equipment, if needed.
—	—	—	7. Turn on the suction unit. Adjust the pressure, if needed, to the level set by unit policy.
—	—	—	8. Position the patient properly for suctioning.
—	—	—	9. Suction the oropharynx of the patient to remove secretions.
—	—	—	10. Rinse the suction tip and tubing in a cup of sterile water or saline solution.
—	—	—	11. Repeat steps 9 and 10 as needed.
—	—	—	12. Note the amount, color, odor, and consistency of the secretions.
—	—	—	13. Monitor the patient's breathing, pulse, and appearance.
—	—	—	14. Report observations to proper health care personnel.
—	—	—	15. Chart as necessary (date, time, procedure, patient condition).
—	—	—	16. After the procedure is completed, return the patient to his or her former position and the room to its normal condition.

DC means done correctly.
DI means done incorrectly. (This step must be repeated and done correctly to complete the checkoff. A note is needed stating the problem and that it was corrected.)
NA means not appropriate. (This step was not needed in this procedure.)

Verbal communication with the patient: ___ satisfactory ___ unsatisfactory ___ not needed. Area(s) needing improvement:

Written communication/charting: ____satisfactory ____ unsatisfactory. Area(s) needing improvement:

_____   _____   _____   _____
Evaluator's signature   Date passed   Student's/Employee's signature   Date passed

If previous attempts were unsatisfactory, the problem(s) must be listed here with the remedial action taken to correct the problem. This must be signed by the evaluator and dated.

PROCEDURE 12 CHECKLIST
OROPHARYNGEAL SUCTIONING

Verbal questions that must be answered correctly before starting the procedure:

1. Identify the possible complication of oropharyngeal suctioning.
2. Identify the equipment needed for oropharyngeal suctioning.
3. What two things could cause a loss of vacuum?
4. What would you do if a patient needed deep tracheal suctioning?

CLINICAL checkoff on the procedure.

DC	DI	NA	
___	___	___	1. Confirm that the physician's order is current and complete.
___	___	___	2. Review the chart for current patient information.
___	___	___	3. Greet the patient, identify yourself, and state your purpose.
___	___	___	4. Confirm the patient's identity on his or her wristband.
___	___	___	5. Wash your hands and put on clean gloves, goggles, and mask according to your unit's policy.
___	___	___	6. Gather and assemble the equipment, if needed.
___	___	___	7. Turn on the suction unit. Adjust the pressure, if needed, to the level set by unit policy.
___	___	___	8. Position the patient properly for suctioning.
___	___	___	9. Suction the oropharynx of the patient to remove secretions.
___	___	___	10. Rinse the suction tip and tubing in a cup of sterile water or saline solution.
___	___	___	11. Repeat steps 9 and 10 as needed.
___	___	___	12. Note the amount, color, odor, and consistency of the secretions.
___	___	___	13. Monitor the patient's breathing, pulse, and appearance.
___	___	___	14. Report observations to proper health care personnel.
___	___	___	15. Chart as necessary (date, time, procedure, patient condition).
___	___	___	16. After the procedure is completed, return the patient to his or her former position and the room to its normal condition.

DC means done correctly.
DI means done incorrectly. (This step must be repeated and done correctly to complete the checkoff. A note is needed stating the problem and that it was corrected.)
NA means not appropriate. (This step was not needed in this procedure.)

Verbal communication with the patient: ___ satisfactory ___ unsatisfactory ___ not needed. Area(s) needing improvement:

Written communication/charting: ____satisfactory ____ unsatisfactory. Area(s) needing improvement:

_____   _____   _____   _____
Evaluator's signature   Date passed   Student's/Employee's signature   Date passed

If previous attempts were unsatisfactory, the problem(s) must be listed here with the remedial action taken to correct the problem. This must be signed by the evaluator and dated.

Chapter 1

Anderson, K. N., ed. *Mosby's Medical, Nursing, & Allied Health Dictionary,* 4th ed. St. Louis: Mosby-Year Book, Inc., 1994.

Des Jardins, T. *Cardiopulmonary Anatomy and Physiology,* 2d ed. Albany, NY: Delmar Publishers, Inc., 1993.

Marieb, E. N. *Human Anatomy and Physiology,* 2d ed. Redwood City, CA: Benjamin/Cummings Publishing, 1992.

Matthews, L. R. *Cardiopulmonary Anatomy and Physiology.* Philadelphia: Lippincott-Raven Publishers, 1996.

Murray, J. F. *The Normal Lung.* Philadelphia: W. B. Saunders, 1986.

Chapter 2

American Heart Association. *Heart and Stroke Facts.* Dallas, TX: American Heart Association, 1994.

Anderson, K. N., ed. *Mosby's Medical, Nursing, & Allied Health Dictionary,* 4th ed. St. Louis: Mosby-Year Book, Inc., 1994.

Bellenir, K., and Dresser, P. D., eds. *Cardiovascular Diseases and Disorders Sourcebook.* Detroit, MI: Omnigraphics, Inc., 1995.

Cook, A. R., and Dresser, P. D., eds. *Respiratory Diseases and Disorders Sourcebook.* Detroit, MI: Omnigraphics, Inc., 1995.

Des Jardins, T. *Clinical Manifestations & Assessment of Respiratory Disease,* 3d ed. St. Louis, MO: Mosby-Year Book, Inc., 1995.

Hamann, B. *Disease: Identification, Prevention, and Control.* St. Louis, MO: Mosby-Year Book, Inc., 1994.

Thomas, C. L., ed. *Taber's Cyclopedic Medical Dictionary,* 18th ed. Philadelphia: F. A. Davis, 1997.

Wilkins, R. L., and Dexter, J. R. *Respiratory Disease: Principles of Patient Care.* Philadelphia: F. A. Davis, 1993.

Chapter 3

American Association for Respiratory Care. Clinical Practice Guideline: Defibrillation During Resuscitation. *Respiratory Care, 40*(7), 744–748 (July 1995).

American Association for Respiratory Care. Clinical Practice Guideline: Directed Cough. *Respiratory Care, 38*(5), 495–499 (May 1993).

American Association for Respiratory Care. Clinical Practice Guideline: Endotracheal Suctioning of Mechanically Ventilated Adults and Children with Artificial Airways. *Respiratory Care, 38*(5), 500–504 (May 1993).

American Association for Respiratory Care. Clinical Practice Guideline: Incentive Spirometry. *Respiratory Care, 36*(12), 1402–1405 (December 1991).

American Association for Respiratory Care. Clinical Practice Guideline: Management of Airway Emergencies. *Respiratory Care, 40*(7), 749–760 (July 1995).

American Association for Respiratory Care. Clinical Practice Guideline: Oxygen Therapy in the Acute Care Hospital. *Respiratory Care, 36*(12), 1410–1413 (December 1991).

American Association for Respiratory Care. Clinical Practice Guideline: Patient-Ventilator System Checks. *Respiratory Care, 37*(8), 882–886 (August 1992).

American Association for Respiratory Care. Clinical Practice Guideline: Postural Drainage Therapy. *Respiratory Care, 36*(12), 1418–1426 (December 1991).

American Association for Respiratory Care. Clinical Practice Guideline: Pulse Oximetry. *Respiratory Care, 36*(12), 1406–1409 (December 1991).

American Association for Respiratory Care. Clinical Practice Guideline: Resuscitation in Acute Care Hospitals. *Respiratory Care, 38*(11), 1179–1188 (November 1993).

American Association for Respiratory Care. Clinical Practice Guideline: Sampling for Arterial Blood Gas Analysis. *Respiratory Care, 37*(8), 913–917 (August 1992).

American Association for Respiratory Care. Clinical Practice Guideline: Selection of Aerosol Delivery Device. *Respiratory Care, 37*(8), 891–897 (August 1992).

Barnes, T. A. *Core Textbook of Respiratory Care Practice,* 2d ed. St. Louis, MO: Mosby-Year Book, Inc., 1994.

Branson, R. D., Hess, D. R., and Chatburn, R. L. *Respiratory Care Management.* Philadelphia: J. B. Lippincott, 1995.

Burton, G. G., Hodgkin, J. E., and Ward, J. J. *Respiratory Care: A Guide to Clinical Practice,* 3d ed. Philadelphia: J. B. Lippincott, 1991.

Dantzker, D. R., MacIntyre, N. R., and Bakow, E. D. *Comprehensive Respiratory Care.* Philadelphia: W. B. Saunders, 1995.

McPherson, S. P. *Respiratory Care Equipment,* 5th ed. St. Louis, MO: Mosby-Year Book, Inc., 1995.

Scanlan, C. L., Spearman, C. B., and Sheldon, R. L. *Egan's Fundamentals of Respiratory Care,* 6th ed. St. Louis, MO: Mosby-Year Book, Inc., 1995.

Sills, J. R. *Respiratory Care Certification Guide,* 2d ed. St. Louis, MO: Mosby-Year Book, Inc., 1994.

Sills, J. R. *Respiratory Care Registry Guide.* St. Louis, MO: Mosby-Year Book, Inc., 1995.

White, G. C. *Equipment Theory for Respiratory Care,* 2d ed. Albany, NY: Delmar Publishers, 1996.